BOB
MARLEY

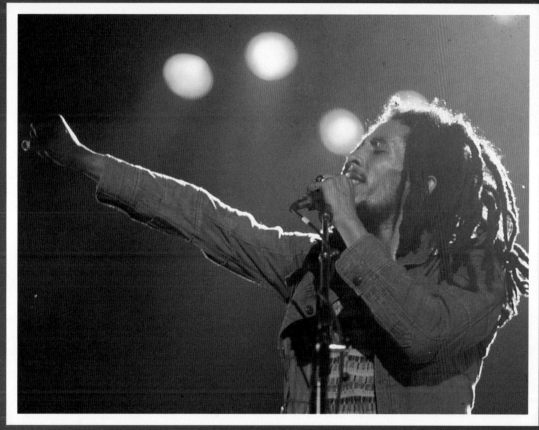

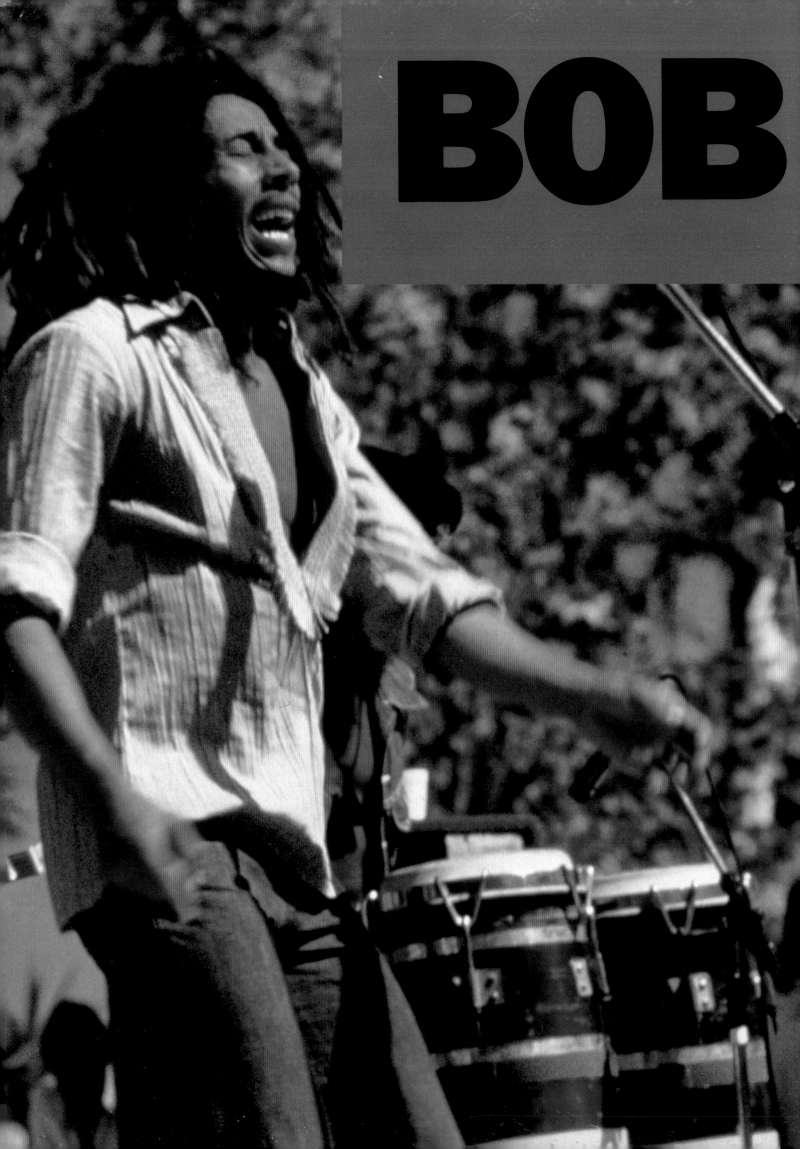

BOB

MARLEY

Margaret E Ward

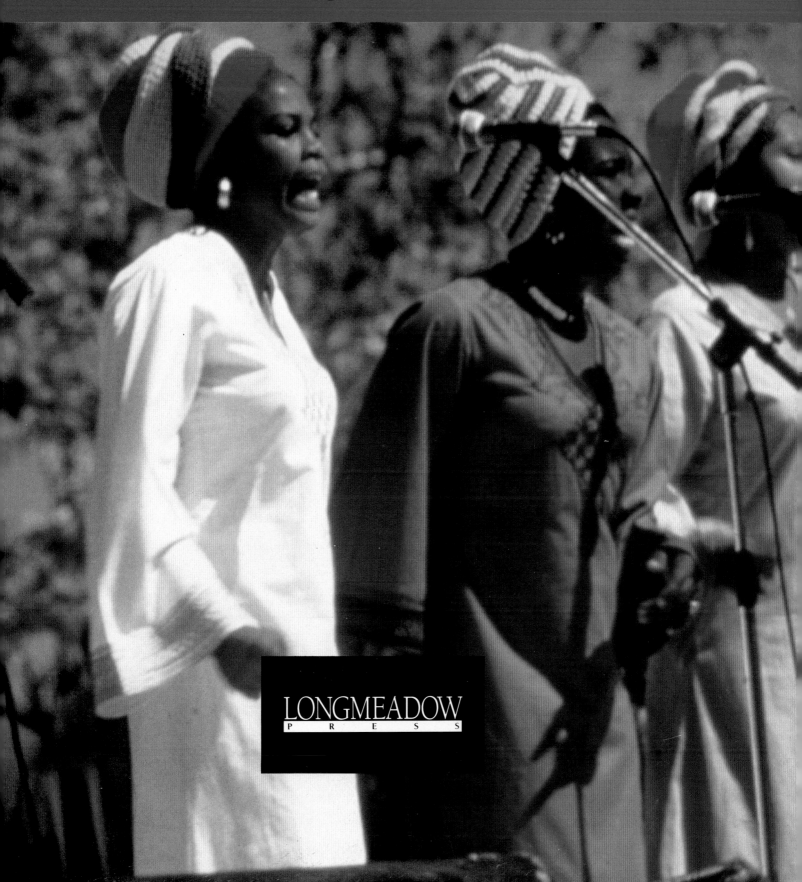

LONGMEADOW
PRESS

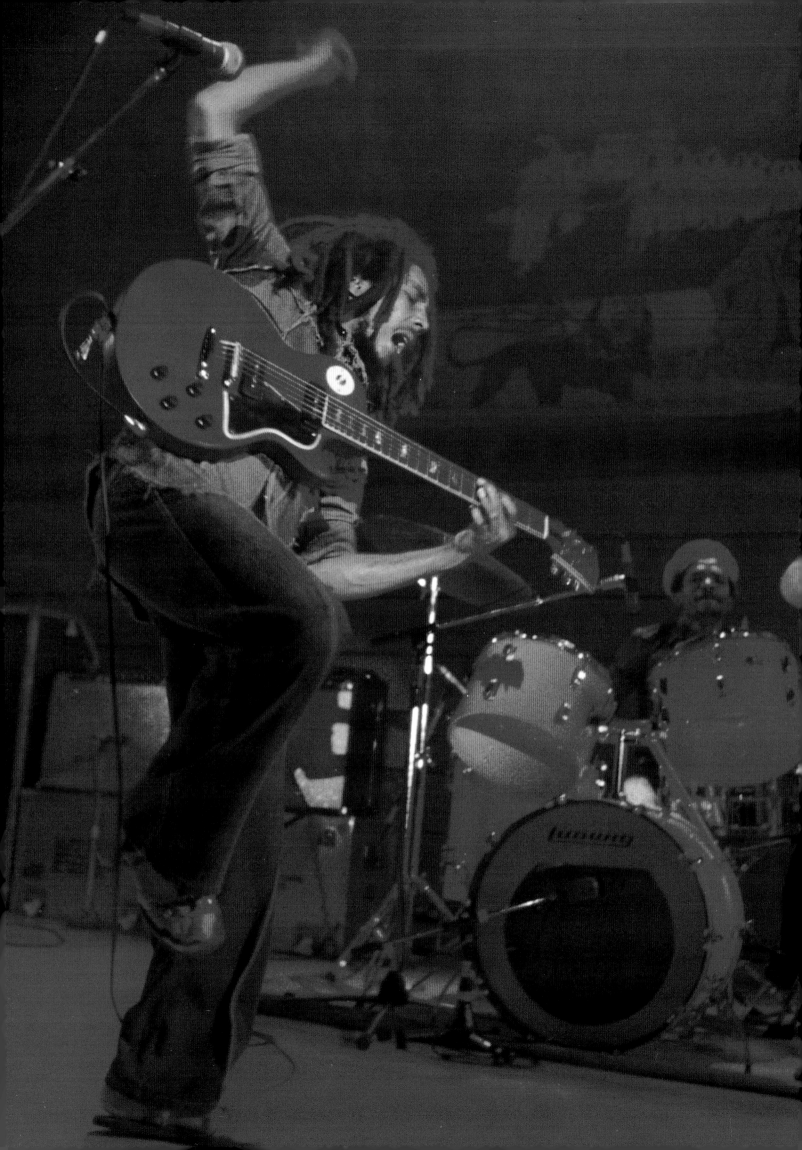

Picture Credits
The Bettmann Archive: page 8.
© *Adrian Boot/Retna Ltd.*: pages 7, 10 (top), 11 (bottom), 26, 27 (right), 41 (top right), 68 (top left), 71, 76 (top left).
British Film Institute: pages 15, 31 (top right).
Claude Gassian: pages 1, 14, 28, 32 (both), 50-51, 53, 58-59, 60-61, 62-63, 64-65, 66, 67 (top left, right), 72-73, 74 (both), 76 (bottom left), 77.
Globe Photos: page 18 (left); *Globe Photos/ Dennis Barna*: page 57; *Globe Photos/ Adrian Boot*: pages 56, 67 (bottom), 75 left).
Jamaican Daily Gleaner: pages 16 (both), 21 (left).
Jampress Ltd., Jamaican Information Service: page 20.
London Features International: pages 24 (top), 30 (bottom right); *LFI/Adrian Boot*: page 37.
© *Mail Newspapers/Solo*: page 68 (bottom left).
© *Bob Marley Foundation/Retna Ltd.*: pages 21 (right), 22, 23 (bottom right), 25 (top).
Michael Ochs Archives: pages 13 (top left), 17, 24 (bottom).
Pictorial Press: pages 2-3, 36, 41 (bottom).
© *Relay Photos/Andre Csillag*: page 27 (top left).
Rex USA: page 29.
© *Kate Simon*: pages 4, 6, 9, 13, 19 (bottom right), 25 (bottom left), 33 (both), 34-35, 38-39, 40, 42 (bottom right), 43 (top right), 44-45, 46-47, 48-49, 52, 54-55, 68 (right), 69, 76 (bottom right), 79.
UPI/Bettmann Newsphotos: pages 10 (bottom), 11 (top), 12 (both), 19 (top left), 23 (top left), 30 (top left), 42 (top left), 70.

This 1993 edition published by Longmeadow Press
201 High Ridge Road
Stamford CT 06904

Produced by
Brompton Books Corporation
15 Sherwood Place
Greenwich CT 06830

ISBN 0-681-41866-4

Printed in Hong Kong

0 9 8 7 6 5 4 3 2 1

Acknowledgments
Irie to my good fairy and editor, Jean Martin, for the opportunity to publish my first book. Peace and love to my cheerleaders, Ami and Kim, whose 'rah, rah's' kept me going. Thanks to my brother Owen, whose many gifts continually inspire me, and my late mother for her spiritual guidance. Many thanks to my reggae friend, Tony Gorman, for his knowledge. Most of all, thanks to Bob Marley for his stirring message.

   Thanks also go to the following people who helped in the preparation of this book: Sara Dunphy, the picture editor; Adrian Hodgkins, the designer; Nicki Giles for production; and Elizabeth A. McCarthy, the indexer.

PAGE 1: **The Rasta prophet in Paris, 1977.**

PAGES 2-3: **Bob Marley and the I-Threes in full cry.**

LEFT: **Bob Marley was known for his mesmerizing performances. Here he is during the *Exodus* tour in 1977.**

THE LION OF JUDAH
1945~61

RIGHT: The photograph used on the *Legend* album cover, the most famous of the Marley portraits.

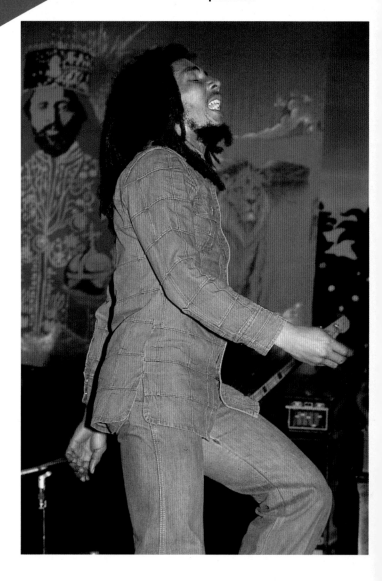

RIGHT: Bob Marley on stage during a European tour, flanked by a portrait of Emperor Haile Selassie I of Ethiopia and a lion.

Bob Marley's dreaded mane shook as he stared in disbelief at the ring that had just been placed on his finger. It fit perfectly, and the gold symbol of the Lion of Judah glittered its reflections into his eyes. Strangely enough, he had dreamt of this moment eleven years before – only differently. He couldn't possibly have imagined that the ring he received in his dream would actually belong to the man he, and other Rastafarians, considered 'Jah' or God.

Emperor Haile Selassie I of Ethiopia, known as the Lion of Judah and 'Jah Rastafari' which means 'lion's head,' had owned this ring. Bob Marley had embraced Rastafarianism in the late 1960s and believed, as they did, that Selassie was the living god, the man who would free them from oppression.

Jamaicans, and Rastafarians in particular, are a people who see power in the spiritual and the symbolic. Bob Marley was no

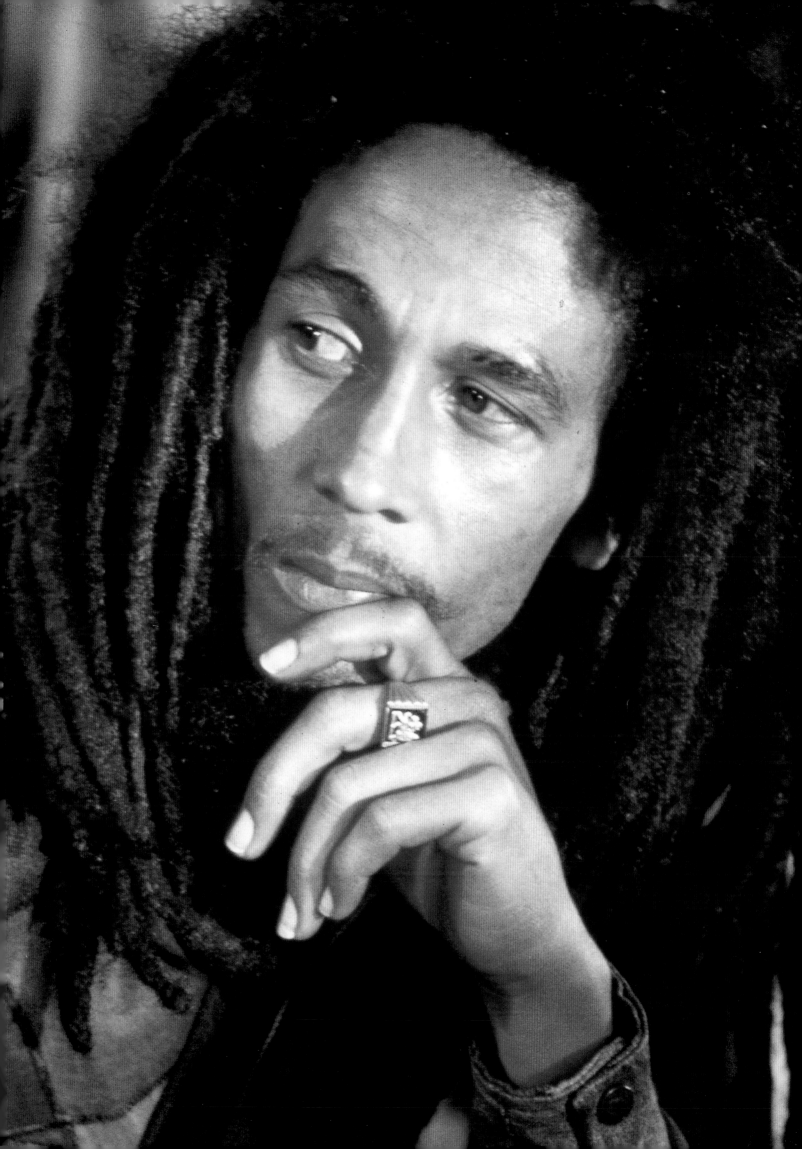

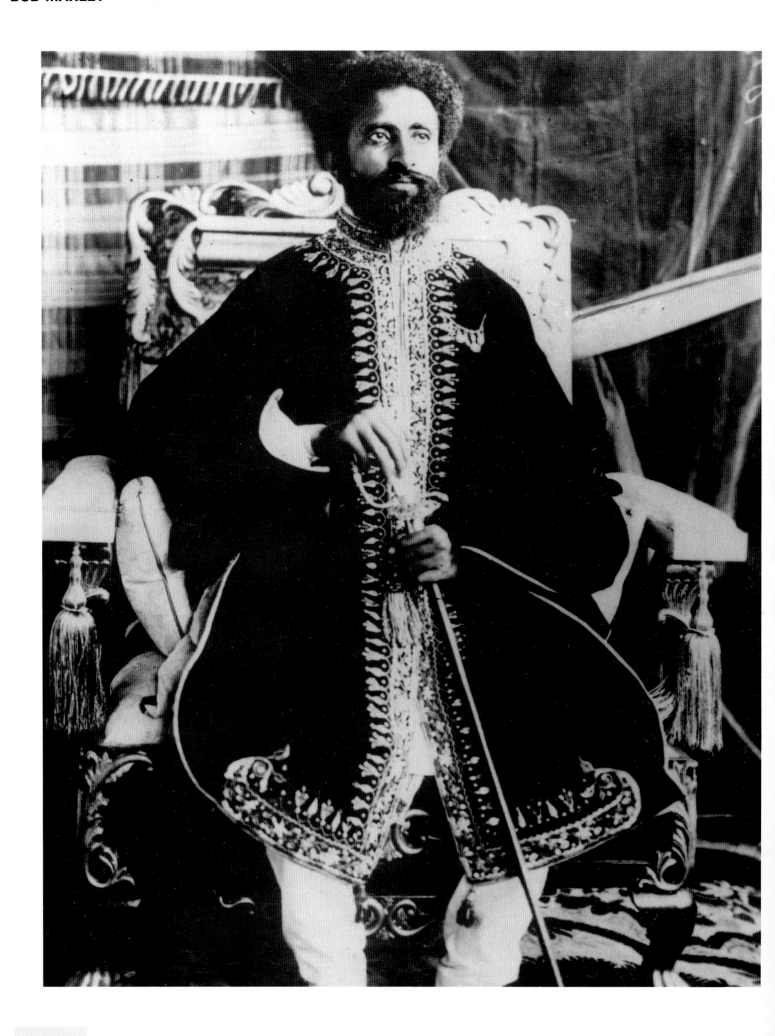

LEFT: **The diminutive, yet larger-than-life Emperor Haile Selassie I at his coronation in 1930. Not as popular with his subjects as he was with Jamaican Rastafarians, Selassie was dethroned and eventually buried in a pauper's grave upon his death in 1975.**

RIGHT: **Bob delivers the Rasta message from his favorite pulpit – the stage.**

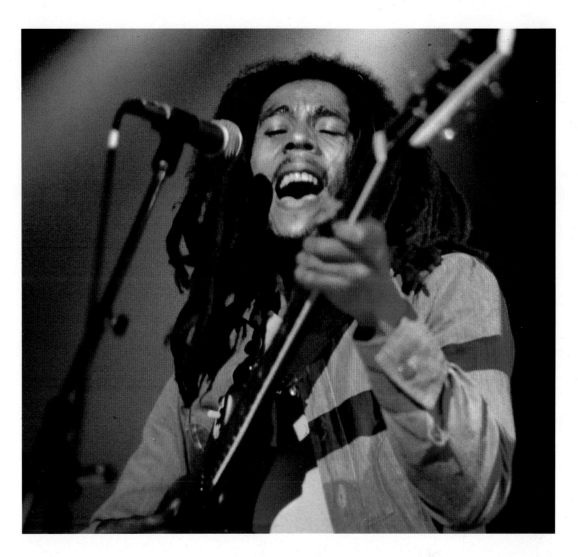

exception. The fact that he received the ring in 1977 is wrought with symbolic significance. According to signs in the scriptures, Rastafarian soothsayers had predicted that 1977 would be a pivotal year for Rastas. Was this the event they had predicted? No one can be sure, but Marley certainly lived by his beliefs and is considered a prophet by many. Marley preached his message of anti-racism, equality and freedom from oppression on every continent during his 19-year career. His lyrics and rebel rhythms contained a forceful message during the racially and politically turbulent 1960s and 1970s. This message has withstood the test of time, and is relevant even today.

A contemplative Marley wears the ring on the cover of *Legend*, an album released in 1984, three years after his death. This album is one of more than 25 albums and hundreds of singles which span his spectacular career.

Bob Marley thrilled audiences with a new type of music, a blend of African beats and American rhythm and blues and soul, known as reggae. Although other artists established the style, Marley was responsible for bringing this new music from the Caribbean island of Jamaica to international audiences. He was a diminutive man at five feet four inches, but he packed a powerful message into his music and surrounded it with a pulsatingly danceable beat.

In 1975, *Rolling Stone* magazine claimed 'Marleymania' was sweeping America. Marley and the Wailers, his original band, played gigs with such 1970s superstars as Stevie Wonder and Sly and the Family Stone. During that same period, Eric Clapton and Johnny Nash recorded some of Bob's compositions, and his music influenced Paul Simon's 'Mother and Child Reunion' album.

Bob Marley mesmerized audiences everywhere. As a performer, he was a firebrand of movement and expression on stage. As a person, he was mysterious and spiritual, considered a Rastafarian prophet by some and an enigma by others.

Bob was different from the very start. He was born Robert Nesta Marley, the child of a young, black Jamaican girl from the countryside and a much older, white, British military man. After he impregnated the young Cedella Malcolm, fifty-year-old Captain Norval Sinclair Marley of the British West India Regiment wed her and then made a hasty departure for Kingston. 'Ciddy' would not see him again until a few months before his death in 1955.

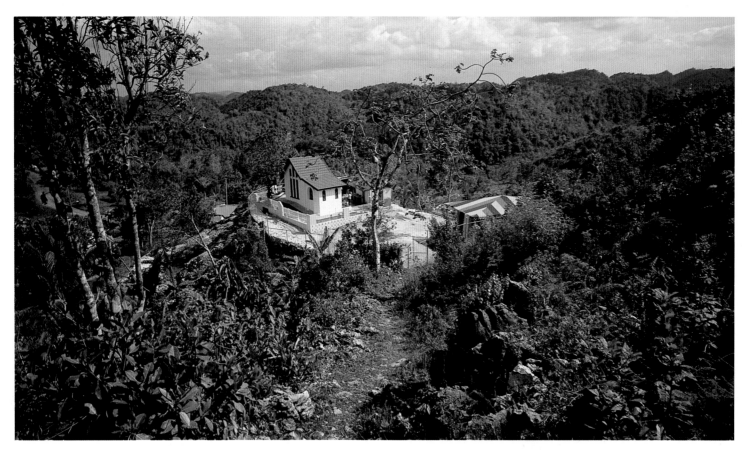

Nesta, as Bob was called at that time, was born on 6 February 1945 in Nine Miles, St Ann parish (or county), Jamaica. Marcus Garvey, another important figure in the Rastafarian movement, had been born in St. Ann 58 years before Marley. Garvey's message strongly influenced Marley's life and work. In simplified terms, Garvey believed in the equality of blacks and the promotion of black pride, a foreign notion at the time. He believed that blacks should be proud of their African heritage and that they should ultimately return to Africa. Garvey predicted that a black king would be born in Africa and liberate the Negro race. To Rastafarians, Haile Selassie I was the fulfilment of that prophecy.

Another strong influence on Bob's life was his grandfather and surrogate father, Omeriah Malcolm. Malcolm was Ciddy's father and a well-respected figure in the rural community. The sizeable Malcolm family lived in the area and worked together to cultivate the land on their large homestead and run several of the family-owned businesses.

In an interview with black American television host Gil Noble in 1980, Marley said that when he lived in the country he learned to rely on family and work hard on the farm. Unfortunately, the togetherness and shelter of country life only lasted five years. He was kidnapped and taken to Kingston by the Captain, his father, and wasn't reunited with Ciddy until a year later.

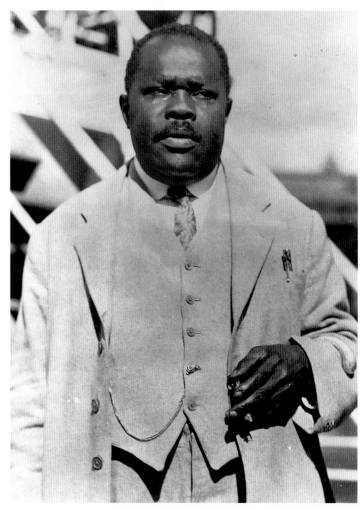

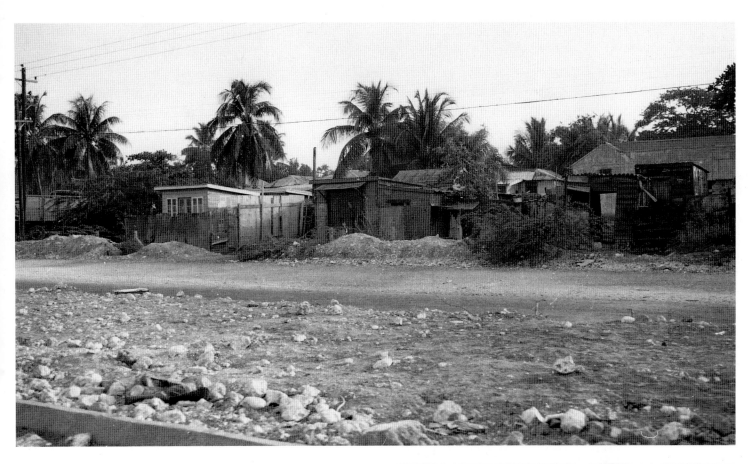

Some years later, in search of work and excitement, Ciddy moved with Bob to Kingston. They lived in Trench Town, one of the most dangerous slums in the capital. Toddy Livingston and his son Bunny, a friend of Bob's, agreed to live with them in one of the 'government yard' apartments. The poorly constructed buildings were originally built as emergency shelters. They later inspired Marley to write a song called 'Concrete Jungle,' which likened the living conditions and poverty in the slum to the shackles of slavery.

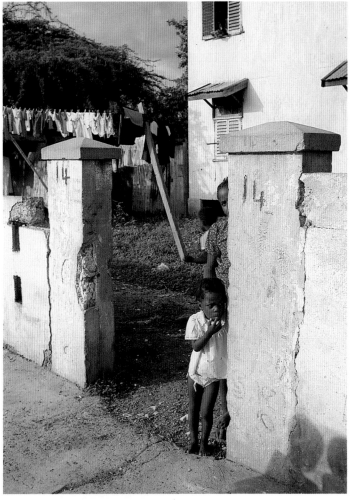

TOP LEFT: **Nine Miles, St. Ann parish, Jamaica, the birthplace of Marcus Garvey and Bob Marley.**

LEFT: **Marcus Mosiah Garvey (1887-1940) was initially scorned in Jamaica for his "black pride" and "back to Africa" beliefs.**

TOP: **One of the many slums in Kingston, Jamaica. Many poor Jamaican teens sought their fortune in the Kingston recording industry but lived and struggled in the mostly black slums.**

RIGHT: **A scene in Trench Town, the slum in Kingston where Bob Marley lived and recorded during his early teens.**

Trench Town, like most slums, was a violent place where gangs often battled it out with knives and guns in broad daylight. Bob and Bunny quickly learned how to survive the tough streets. They became street fighters, or 'rude bwais,' and masterful players of soccer, a favorite Jamaican sport. Bob eventually earned the ghetto nickname, Tuff Gong.

The 'rush-rush' of city life appealed to Bob and so did the music he was hearing. It was the late 1950s, and Jamaicans listened to US radio stations for all the popular songs from such musicians as Fats Domino, Ray Charles, Brook Benton and Curtis Mayfield. New Orleans jazz and rhythm and blues, usually performed by black musicians, heavily influenced most of the music at that time.

At the same time, Jamaican musicians were busily working on musical hybrids of their own. In the early 1960s, ska was the most predominant of these forms in Jamaica. It combined the catchy back beat of New Orleans-style R&B and Jamaican mento, a type of calypso music. Ska music accented the second and fourth beats and the back beat was played on a piano or rhythm guitar. It soon became a dancehall sensation.

As Bob and Bunny entered their teens they began to go to 'jump-ups,' or local dances featuring ska music. The dances were held by local record shop owners who placed mega-watt amplifiers in the yards or in villages. Not only did the hand-picked DJs promote the latest releases for the record store, but the owners also made a hefty profit by charging admission to the extremely popular events. Usually, the sound system was attached to a van or truck and the DJs travelled around to promote the hottest singles and to compete with their rivals. It was an ingenious way to bring music to people who couldn't afford the luxury of a radio but could scrape together a few shillings to hear their favorite hits.

Bob, like many Jamaican teenagers, found music a relief from the realities of ghetto life. All youths were looking for way out of the endless cycle of poverty. Crime was a solution for some, known as 'rudies,' but it almost certainly ended in an early death on the violent Kingston streets.

Bob dreamed of music while attending school. However, schoolwork prepared him for big dreams which would only result in empty solutions. The menial life he was destined for in Trench Town had nothing to do with algebra and science. By the time he was 15 he stopped his schooling, and became a welder's apprentice. At least this way he could bring some money into the household.

Ska spread like a fever through the restless teenage masses, and Bob was easily distracted from his welding work as he

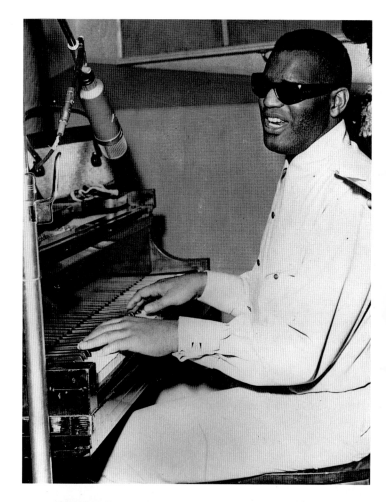

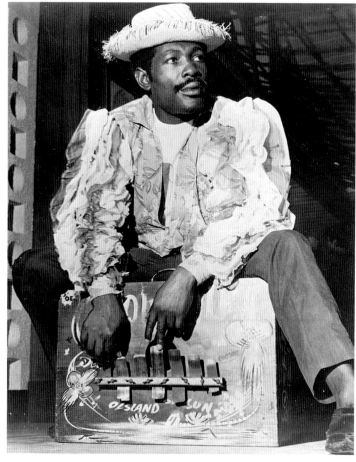

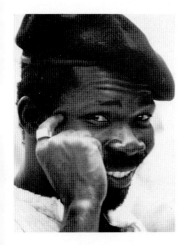

ABOVE: Joe Higgs, the man who taught the young Marley the tricks of the trade. He later joined the Wailers during the 1973 US tour, replacing Bunny Livingston.

LEFT: Ray Charles, American singer and musician, was one of Marley's major early influences.

RIGHT: Bob playing the guitar in Paris, 1977.

BELOW LEFT: A typically costumed Calypso singer plays the Jamaican marimba box, which sounds like a piano. Calypso gradually gave way to ska and reggae as the dominant sounds in Jamaica.

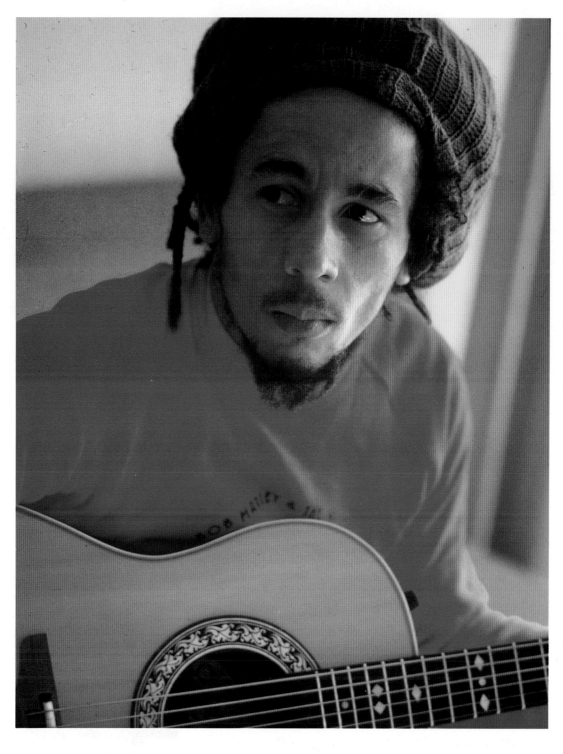

concentrated on mastering the new ska harmonies. While welding one day, a piece of burning hot metal flew into his eye and ended his welding career. He told his mother he was actually relieved, because it meant he could spend more time on his recording career. His intentions were considered foolhardy, since at that time everyone wanted to be a recording star.

The 'youts,' as Bob called the people he grew up with in the Kingston slums, were drawn towards a charismatic Rastafarian called Joe Higgs. A couple of years back, Bob had recorded a few singles with a new producer named Edward Seaga for the

WIRL label, and they had been big hits. Higgs held free music clinics at his home on Third Street, only a street away from Bob's home. Coached by the perfectionist Higgs, teenagers would harmonize through the night, with occasional breaks for a bit of fruit or goat. Through most of the day, many of the children would sing to stave off their hunger pangs.

At 16, Marley was hungry for his first record. Little did he know that his recording career would lead him on a spiritual journey and make him the Third World's first international superstar.

SIMMER DOWN
1962-67

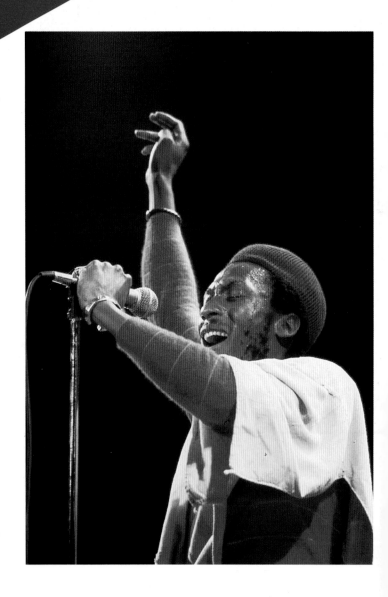

Jimmy Cliff on stage (BELOW) **and as Rhyging in** *The Harder They Come* **(1973)** (RIGHT).

In 1962, the restlessness in the ghetto was reflective of the turmoil taking place in the Jamaican government. Two rival political parties, the Jamaican Labor Party (JLP) and the People's National Party (PNP) were gearing up for one of many knock-down, drag-out fights.

In the streets, a 'rude bwai' named Vincent 'Ivanhoe' Martin had become a legend. His ability to out-maneuver the police had caught the imagination of the oppressed poor, who called him 'Rhyging,' meaning angry. Jimmy Cliff, a local musician, would later immortalize Rhyging in his 1973 film *The Harder They Come*. It was this film which first brought reggae to the United States.

All over Kingston, tensions were high, and the early 1960s marked the beginning of nearly two decades of political strife and police harassment of the poor in Jamaica. In order to escape their frustrations, people were increasingly turning towards music to express themselves. Everyone in the yards and tenements wanted to make a record. Many record shop owners had become music producers by utilizing Kingston's various recording studios. Leslie Kong owned the Beverley's record label and a store by the same name. Clement Seymour 'Sir Coxsone' Dodd of sound system fame, owned Musik City and produced labels under the names World Disk, Coxsone, Musik City, Studio One and D Darling.

Bob had been diligently working away on songs he planned to show one of the producers. During his welding apprenticeship, he had become friends with Desmond Dekker, who had just made a recording with Count Boysie, another local producer, at Federal Studios.

By this time, 14-year-old Jimmy Cliff had released several singles, the most recent of which, 'Miss Jamaica,' was doing well.

Cliff said during an interview following a World Beat '92 Tour performance:

'It was in Kingston that I met Bob at Leslie Kong, who was my t'ird producer. Bob was brought to me by Desmond Dekker. Bob wanted to start his recording career and I already had probably two, t'ree years into my (sic) to establish myself. Bob wanted to get started, so that was his start.

'He just came with his songs and I was playing the piano. I said, "Sing the songs," he sang, I played. I played them and I feel them sounded good and I took him to the producer [Leslie Kong]. That was his start. He was alone at the time, he didn't have any Wailers or anybody.

'We went to the studio and three weeks later we recorded these songs: "Judge Not," "One Cup of Coffee," and "Terror."'

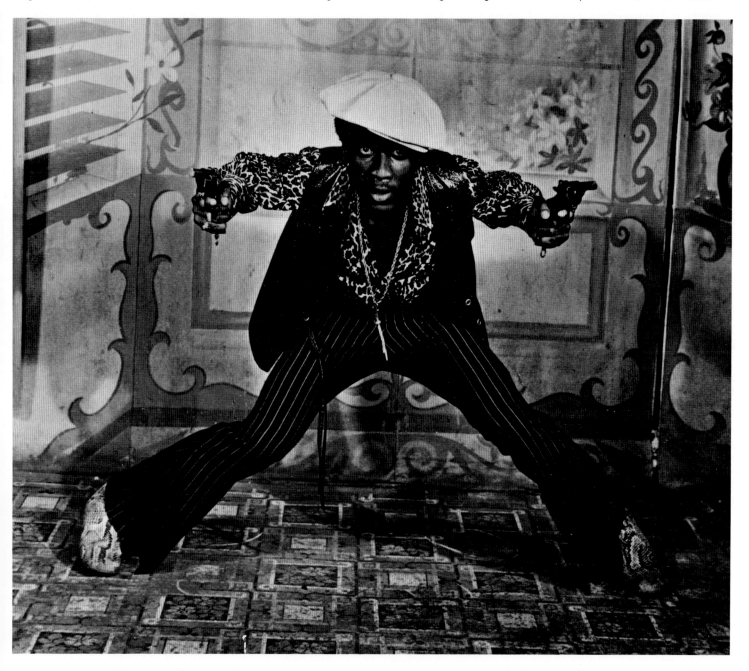

Apparently, Marley was fairly confident during that recording session. Cliff said, 'He [Bob] was a sensitive guy. He was always a very sensitive guy. He just came in and I was playing, he didn't seem nervous at the time.'

'Judge Not' with a B-side of 'Do You Still Love Me' (recorded later) was released as Marley's first single. Due to a typographical error, the record was released under the name Bob Morley. But if Leslie Kong had had his way that day, Bob Marley wouldn't have been Bob Marley at all, according to Jimmy Cliff:

'Leslie Kong wanted to change his name to call him Haddam. He didn't want to change. I tell him to keep his name. At the time in Jamaica, you look for a name that sounds commercial, or somebody can call easy. Bob Marley don't sound like a name that would be, or obert, didn't sound like a name that sound like a stage name. But, Haddam!'

Bob recorded more singles for Kong, but went his own way after Kong refused to pay him for them. While Marley was deciding what to do next, he returned to Higgs's Trench Town sessions.

After a few sessions, Bob quickly pulled a group together to show Higgs. It included Bunny, Peter McIntosh (later shortened to Tosh), Junior Braithwaite and two female backup singers,

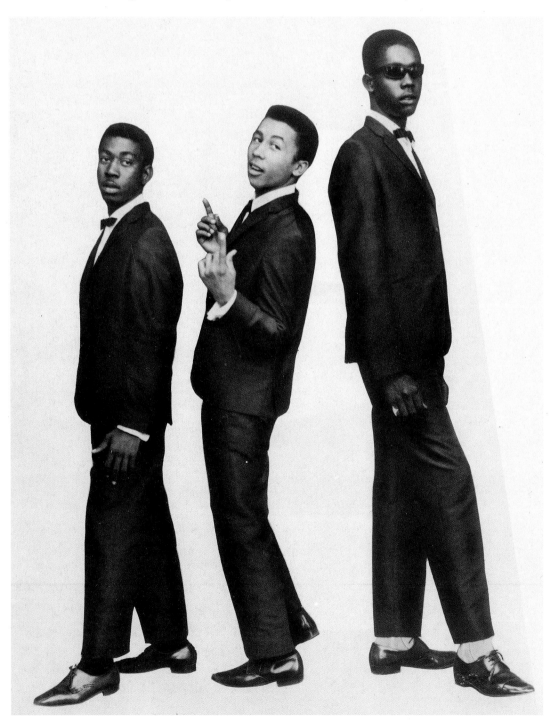

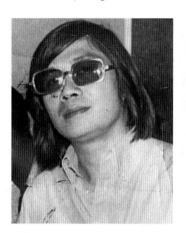

ABOVE: **Shrewd Chinese-Jamaican businessman Leslie Kong gave Marley his first big break.**

LEFT: **An early ska-style publicity shot of the Wailers. Left to right: Bunny Livingston, Bob Marley and Peter Tosh.**

FAR RIGHT, ABOVE: **Ska, jazz and mento guitar legend Ernest Ranglin. His first international recognition as a ska guitarist came with the US hit 'My Boy Lollipop' in 1964. Rod Stewart played harmonica and Millie Small provided the vocals.**

Beverley Kelso and Cherry Smith. Higgs took an interest in the group and coached them exhaustively. After Higgs was picked up by Coxsone, he arranged an audition for the fledgling group. Dodd liked them and they began to record some ska tunes for his labels.

Cherry and Junior left the group after only a few recording sessions, leaving Bob, Bunny, Peter and Beverley. The group went by a variety of names which included 'The Wailers,' 'The Wailing Wailers,' 'Peter Touch and the Wailers,' and 'Bob Marley and the Wailers,' and over the next three years they recorded more than 75 tracks for Coxsone.

'Simmer Down,' a Wailers' track which featured the famous ska guitarist Ernest Ranglin and his group the Skatalites, hit Number One in February 1964. It was their first hit. Bob had been responsible for the lyrics and lead vocals. While the song was still considered ska, it was unusual because the lyrics dealt directly with life in the ghetto, and in particular with 'rude bwais.'

Dodd, riding the popularity of 'Simmer Down,' soon released more Wailers' tracks on the Studio One label, including 'It Hurts to Be Alone' and 'I'm Still Waiting,' which were among some of the earliest tracks the group laid down for him. They continued to produce hits for Dodd's various labels, and he set them up with live gigs in Kingston.

The 1964 World's Fair was to be held in New York City and would feature a delegation from Jamaica. Edward Seaga, Higgs's original producer, had recently been appointed Minister of Development and Finance. He was responsible for choosing the entertainment 'ambassadors,' and Jimmy Cliff was one of those chosen to attend. It was probably the first time ska, still a relatively new musical form, was promoted to an international audience.

In the meantime, the Wailers, dressed in flashy gold lamé stage costumes, were dazzling Kingston audiences with their latest compositions. Bob was slowly becoming more comfortable taking over the leads, but was beginning to display the broodingly distant onstage persona which drew the crowds to him even more. He was becoming a Jamaican James Dean, mysterious and inaccessible.

In the fall of that same year, two of the most influential people in Bob's life were buried. The first, his grandfather, Omeriah Malcolm died of cancer and was buried near the family homestead, which he left to Bob. The second, a man whose work was soon to influence Marley, Marcus Garvey, was to be reburied. Garvey's body was transported from England where it had been for 24 years, and was interred in Jamaica. Politically, this was a way for Edward Seaga and the JLP to gain favor with Rastafarians, who were gaining influence on the island.

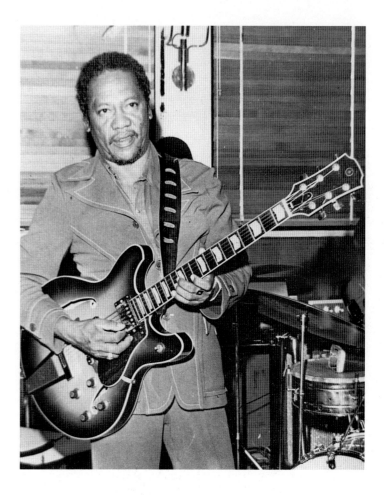

The Wailers enjoyed their popularity through 1965, playing to packed audiences in every arena they played. At times, the overcrowding erupted in violence and the incidents marred the Wailers' reputation in Kingston. It was a year punctuated by brutal race rioting, and by the end of the year the area promoters didn't want to take any chances on the 'rowdy' element the group attracted.

By this time, Rita Anderson had befriended the Wailers. She was a member of the Soulettes, a fledgling Kingston female vocal trio. Bob was unusually shy around her, and through the aid of a note she understood why. He was in love with her. She returned his affections.

Since early 1963, Bob had lived in the streets or in the back of Coxsone's recording studio. His mother had moved to Delaware and other arrangements hadn't worked out. Bob had a bad time trying to sleep at the studio, and one night Rita stayed with him. She awoke gasping for air and fell off the makeshift bed onto the floor. It felt like someone was trying to strangle her. Bob woke up, and saw the now retching Rita. He immediately understood what was happening. Once he took her outside and cleaned her off, he explained he had been taunted by 'duppies,' or spirits of the dead, every night at the studio. That's why he had been unable to sleep.

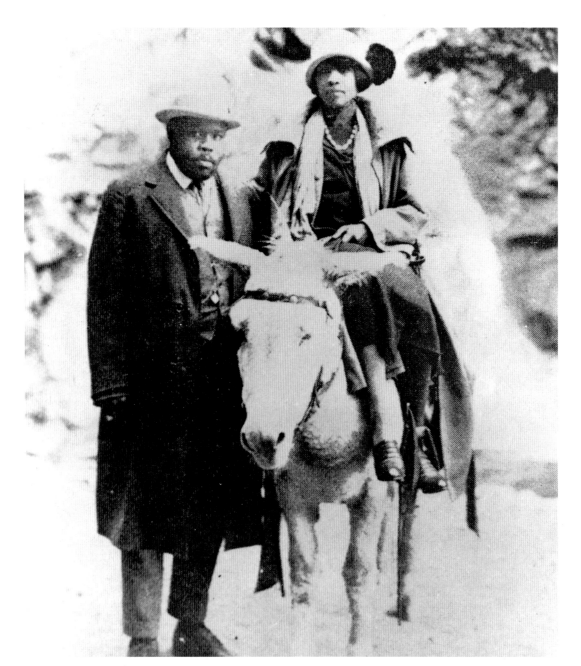

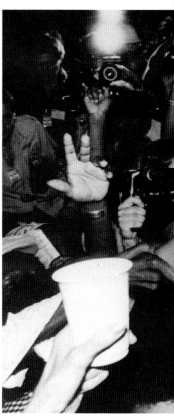

LEFT: **Marcus Garvey, known as the Black Moses, and his second wife Amy Jacques Garvey.**

Rita, who was an equally superstitious Jamaican, was horrified at the situation. The next night she snuck Bob into her room at her aunt's house where she was living while her parents were working abroad. Her aunt, who was extremely disgruntled when she found the sleeping pair, was later convinced that Bob's intentions were honorable. She built a shack for him at the back of their home.

The two eventually married on 10 February 1966. The next day, Bob was on a plane to visit his mother in Delaware where she lived with Edward Booker, her second husband. Prior to that, Ciddy had written Bob several times asking him to come visit her in the United States, but he still went with some reluctance. She wanted him to settle there, but he was itchy to get back to the Wailers, so he only stayed seven months.

While he was away, Beverley quit and Rita and her cousin Dream, or Vision, began singing with the Wailers. Dodd liked the new material and the crowds didn't seem to notice the difference, so they kept playing and recording under the same name. In 1966, Coxsone released the singles 'Love and Affection/Teenager in Love,' 'And I Love Her/Do It Right,' and 'Zimmerman/Lonesome Track' on his Ska Beat label.

Popular music in Jamaica was slowly changing to rock steady, which emphasized less of the exploits of the 'rude bwai' and more of the lover. The rhythm also slowed down to capture a more sensual sound.

Rastafarians were still a misunderstood but growing group in Jamaica. In accordance with their scriptures, they wore their hair in dreadlocks, or long, winding strips resembling rope. Many were still singled out for brutality by the police, and a law required that schoolchildren cut their locks before they were admitted to class.

Hoping to bring national understanding to their cause, the Rasta elders asked Haile Selassie I to visit Jamaica in 1966 and he complied. On 21 April 1966 Selassie was greeted by an estimated 100,000 Rastafarians. The event confirmed what the government had feared: Rastafarians were not just a cult with a tiny following. However, the peacefulness of the event left a good impression on many Jamaicans who were originally fearful of the large turnout. Never before had one person captured the attention of so many of Jamaica's poor.

Rita Marley was raised a Christian, like Bob, and she also taught Sunday school. However, she had heard a great deal about Selassie from fellow musicians who were Rastafarians. She was curious and decided to go see for herself. Rita's curiosity resulted in conversion. Rita wrote Bob in Delaware that she believed she had seen the stigmata, or nail marks of Christ, on Selassie's hands as he drove down the parade route from the airport.

Three months after Selassie's visit, the government's fear of the new movement among the poor resulted in the destruction of

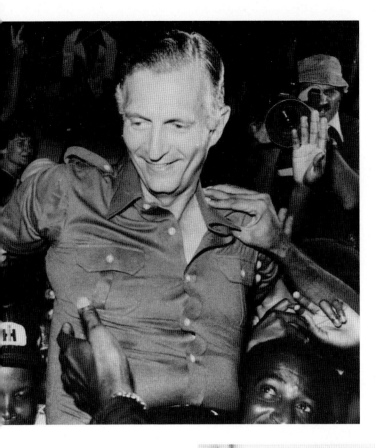

ABOVE: American-born Edward Seaga, record producer (WIRL) turned Jamaican prime minister.

RIGHT: Bob's wife Rita (left) and his mother Ciddy were both raised as Christians and eventually converted to Rastafarianism.

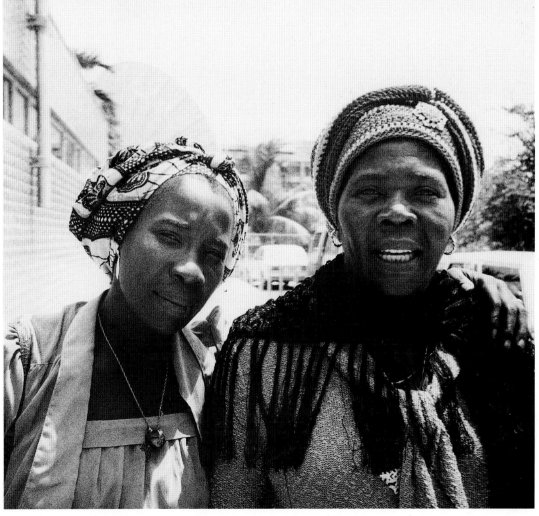

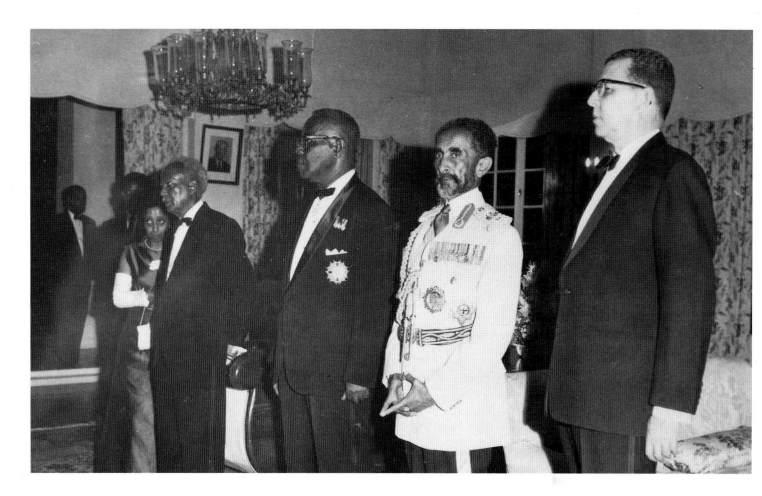

the Back O' Wall squatters' camp. It was an area where thousands lived, mainly Rastas, and they were forced onto the already crowded Kingston streets.

Bob returned from Delaware later that year. Although he was in the United States during Selassie's visit, Bob was deeply influenced by Rita's experience and began asking Rastas about their beliefs. Many musicians in Jamaica, mostly from the lower classes, had already embraced the Rasta way. Bunny had been a Rasts since 1963, and now Bob and Peter allowed their hair and beards to grow in the Rasta fashion.

Coxsone Dodd was less than pleased with the Wailers' conversion and the new direction their music was taking. While Bob was away, Bunny and Peter had several arguments with Dodd about his stinginess. The Wailers and Dodd parted company in 1967 after the Coxsone-produced 'Bend Down Low' was a hit and the group wasn't compensated properly for it.

Bob had already begun to turn away from the ska formula before he left for the United States, with the release of the society-conscious single, 'Simmer Down.' While in Delaware, he worked on the less anxious 'Bend Down Low.' Rock steady was blooming in Kingston and its slower beat allowed people to concentrate on lyrics with meaning. Bob was ready for a new direction when he got back to the island, and it seemed that

his spiritual and musical paths were about to coincide.

After speaking with Joe Higgs, who was a Rasta, Marley sought out Mortimmo Planno, the highest ranking Jamaican Rasta. At first, a confidant for the group, he soon took on an informal managerial role. During this period, Bob was exposed to the traditional drumming and prayer sessions held high in the Jamaican hills. The use of the drums is based on African tribal traditions. The fundeh, bass, and repeater are the three drums usually played during these sessions, which help accent the biblical stories or prayers.

Bob, a natural storyteller, could not help but be influenced by these prayer sessions and the hypnotic beats produced by using drums in that manner. Rock steady's newly focused bass lines, combined with these powerful drums, would begin to allow Bob to show his true writing abilities.

After leaving Coxsone, the Wailers formed a record label called Wail 'N Soul 'M Records (aka Wailing Souls, Wail 'M Soul 'M). The first single put out on the label was 'Bend Down Low/ Mellow Mood.' It had a special tri-colored label which was green, gold and red – the Rasta colors. Bob also turned the shack at the back of Rita's aunt's house at 18 Greenwich Park Road into a record store. The record shack was usually run by Rita and was full of Wailers and Soulettes 45s.

LEFT: **A nervous Haile Selassie 1 was overwhelmed by the throngs of people who greeted him upon his arrival in Jamaica in 1966.**

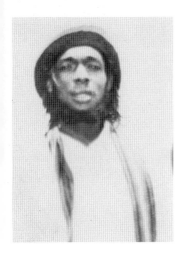

ABOVE: **The elusive, seldom photographed Mortimmo Planno was Bob's first spiritual guide.**

RIGHT: **Peter Tosh (left), Rita and Bob in 1966.**

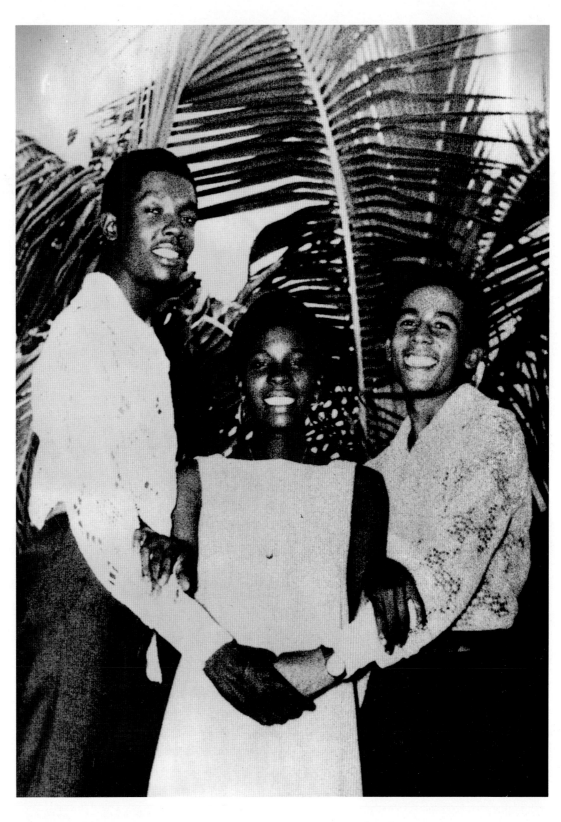

In mid-1967 Bob and Rita, still newlyweds, moved back to the Malcolm homestead in Nine Miles, St Ann parish. It was a time of contemplation and insight for Bob. He spent a great deal of time reading the Bible and working the land. He was returning to his roots for some answers.

Their first child, Cedella, was born that same year. The Marleys started writing together, and some rock steady tunes from these collaborations would eventually emerge on the Wail 'N Soul 'M label. After scraping together some cash, the Wailers recorded two more singles in the fall of that year: 'Hypocrite/ Pound Get a Blow,' and 'Thank You Lord/Nice Time.' The Wailers' music was still popular at jump-ups, but without proper distribution, it never received air time. The label folded at the end of the year.

DUPPY CONQUEROR
1968-71

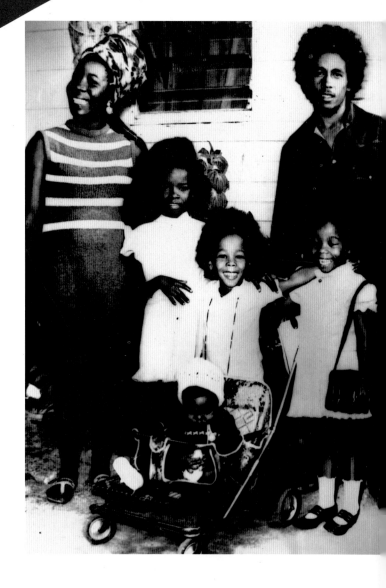

By the end of 1967, Bob had completely embraced 'Jah,' and it was now time for him to put his 'duppies' in order. As a Rastafarian, it was his duty to replace the primitive superstitions of the people with the message of the Lion of Judah. Part of the appeal of the Rastafarian movement for the poor blacks of Kingston was that it encouraged pride in their color and African heritage.

Marley was both black and white and had been scorned by both races. Bob and Ciddy had been abandoned by Bob's father because his family didn't approve of a black 'taint' in the bloodlines. As a young boy growing up in an all-black slum, Bob's thin lips and pointy nose had given away his father's identity as a white man.

Every black Jamaican carried the 'duppies' of self-loathing from the slavery days in Jamaica. Blacks developed a protective

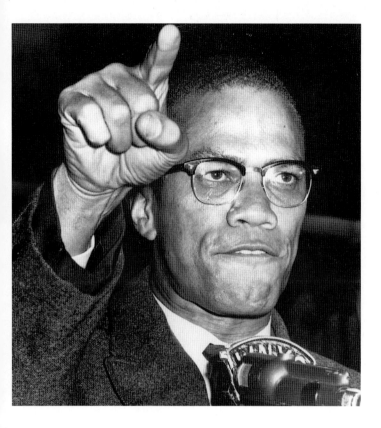

of marijuana, which is illegal in Jamaica but is used sacramentally by the Rastas. Bunny was in jail for the whole year and, needless to say, it was not an active recording year for the group. Bob's first son, David or 'Ziggy,' was born that year.

Before the arrests, Planno was helping the Wailers arrange studio sessions and transportation and advising them on career tactics. But in 1968, they were considered untouchables in the music world and Bob decided to concentrate on learning the Rasta way through Planno.

Marley quickly learned that Rasta was not a religion, but a way of life. He learned that Rastas eat 'ital' food, or food which is pure, free of chemicals and balanced for good health. No salt is consumed, pork is strictly forbidden and the foods are fresh and indigenous to the surrounding countryside. Most Rastas are vegetarian, although some eat fish. They also use local herbs and plants for medicinal purposes and to spice their foods. These dietary laws are geared to promote independence from traditional

character during that period called 'quashie.' The term describes a self-deprecating attitude and way of carrying oneself. In the time of slavery, which was abolished in Jamaica in 1834, pride was not something that was rewarded. Despite the nearly 125 years since slavery was abolished, the 'quashie' remained.

While the Rastas were encouraging black pride in Jamaica, two opposing groups in the US were helping shape the American 'Black Pride' movement. Both wanted racial equality, one through peaceful means and the other 'by any means necessary.' Martin Luther King Jr, and John and Robert Kennedy headed up the peaceful civil rights movement while the Black Panthers, Stokely Carmichael and Malcolm X figured as central characters in the more militant movement.

In 1968, all three Wailers served jail terms for the possession

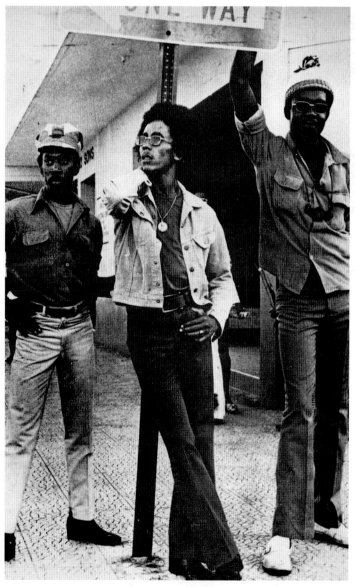

LEFT: Bob, Rita and the first four of their brood. From left to right: Sharon, David 'Ziggy,' Cedella and baby Stephanie in 1972.

TOP: Malcolm X, the militant Muslim spokesman for black pride, at a Harlem rally in 1963.

RIGHT: One way to black pride and equality: The Wailers strike a powerful pose in this photograph taken in Trench Town in 1967 or 1968.

BOB MARLEY

society and give the community the ability to live for extended periods from the land. In giving the people the self-reliance of completely providing for themselves it increases their self esteem and pride.

External adaptations are also essential to the way of life. The brethren and sistren (or brother and sister Rastafari) are encouraged to use 'Rasta talk' as opposed to the colonial English spoken by government officials and the formally educated of Jamaica. The most noticeable physical difference of course has to do with hair. Men grow dreadlocks in accordance with the scriptures and women are required to shave their heads or cover them.

Rastafarians are a very communal people who pray together and provide for the community at large. Education is considered an essential part of the culture and they are usually well-educated in the history of Jamaica and Africa. But Rastafari did not believe in an education which would alienate them from their country's society. So, the children attended regular schools but often were forced to comply with a national law that forced them to be 'properly groomed,' or shave their dreads.

Rastafarian women have a limited role in the society. Usually they are separated from the men and they are responsible for the cooking, childbearing and rearing, and fire-building.

In order to bring them closer to 'Jah' or God, Rastas smoke marijuana. The 'ganja' is smoked from a chillum pipe, a clay water pipe with a straight six-inch stem, or in large cigarettes called 'spliffs.'

In every way, their diet, smoking marijuana, growing dreads, speaking in Rasta talk and living on the fringes of civilization, the Rasta stood out. Most Rasta were also from the poorest segments of society. The government was alarmed at the growing Rasta population and its outspokenness and encouragement of resistance to traditional ways. They had become advocates of the poor and could possibly incite the masses to demand better conditions. As a result they were considered insurgents and were watched carefully.

Musically, a new form had been christened. In a 1992 interview, Toots Hibbert of Toots and the Maytals said: 'When I just started, it wasn't reggae. I'm the one who heard the music and said "Let's do the Reggay" (sic).' That phrase, 'Do the Reggay' was the title of Hibbert's 1968 hit which is said to be responsible for the term.

During a Rasta prayer ceremony, or 'groundation,' that year, Bob met a young, black American performer named Johnny Nash. Nash was impressed with some of the tunes Rita and Bob played for him later in the evening. Later, Nash and his slick promoter, Danny Sims, hired the Wailers as songwriters. Once

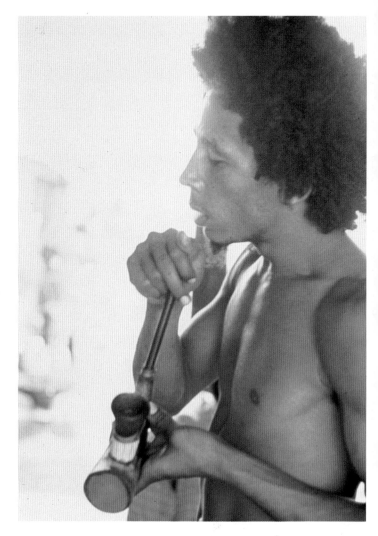
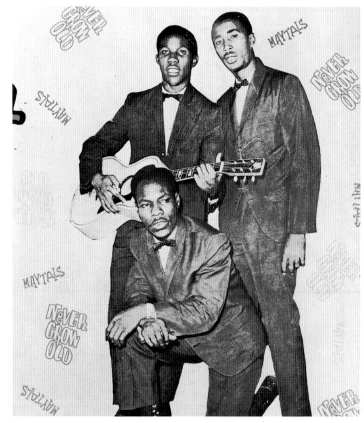

LEFT: **Bob takes a 'toke' of ganja on the sacramental chillum pipe.**

RIGHT: **Dreaded, intense Marley and his cohorts: The Wailers circa 1969-70.**

BOTTOM LEFT: **Toots and the Maytals in the 1960s. Although Toots Hibbert (right) claims he coined the term 'reggae,' others claim the beat named itself.**

BELOW: **Legendary Jamaican record producer Lee 'Scratch' Perry's famous ear and off-beat style helped define the Wailers' sound.**

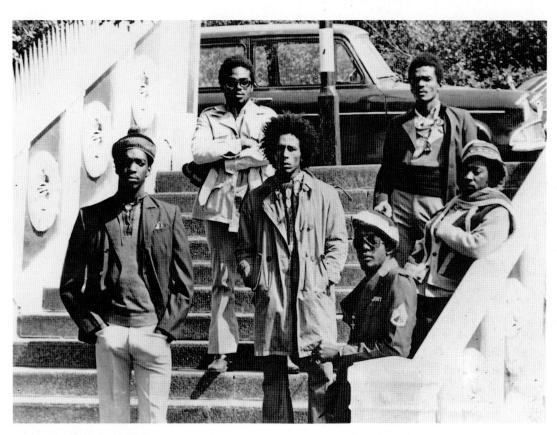

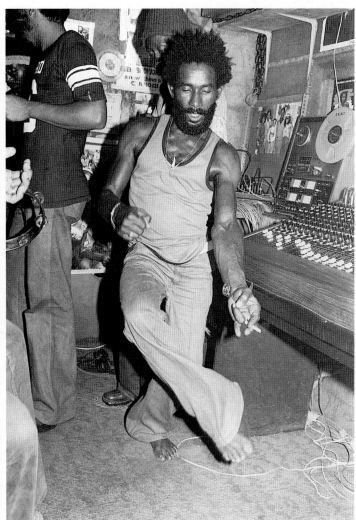

Bunny was out of prison, the Wailers began recording samples of the songs they had written for JAD Records. They continued to produce songs and demos for the company for the next four years.

They were temporarily released from their commitment in 1969 so that they could record a few singles for Leslie Kong. In order to save his family from hunger, Bob had forgiven the producer's monetary indiscretions in the early 1960s.

Reggae was an energetically established form by now and two of the more seductive cuts for Kong were 'Back Out' and 'Do It Twice.' Kong released some of the 45s in Jamaica and in England according to the Wailers' contract with JAD. The singles did poorly and the Wailers were outcasts once again. A year later, much to the chagrin of the group, Kong released the album *The Best of the Wailers*. It made him a millionaire but he didn't live long enough to enjoy it. He died soon afterwards, fulfilling a prophecy Bob had made early in his career. In 1963, he had told a bemused Kong that they would work together again but that Kong would never enjoy any profits from it.

Marley continued to work on his writing and began to invoke the imagery of the Jamaican people. His music was becoming intensely Jamaican. The terminology and visual images in his lyrics were coming from the slang of the ghetto and the folklore of the countryside. Since Marley was from both, it was an extension of his personal experience. In using what was familiar to the people,

Marley carved out new legends, new ways of thinking positively and triumphing over the 'duppies' and old 'Screwface,' or the devil. Two songs which emerged from such imagery and Marley's newly-found spirituality were 'Duppy Conquerer' and 'Screwface.' Both assert Bob's new freedom through his beliefs.

It was just such off-beat imagery that appealed to Lee 'Scratch' Perry, the renegade Coxsone mix-master turned producer. Scratch was actually the one who ended up producing the above two songs. He became the essential piece in the Wailers' sound identity puzzle. Reggae music was filled with heavy bass lines and drums, and Perry felt that Bob's singing hadn't been hard enough against the sounds. With the help of his studio musicians, appropriately called the Upsetters, Perry turned the spit-shined Wailers into a hard-edged, dread machine. Bob and Scratch gave the Wailers the words and the Upsetters gave them souls of rebellion. Some songs released on the Upsetters label from the 1969-70 sessions with Perry include 'Mr Brown,' 'Small Axe,' and 'African Herbsman.' These tracks as well as later recordings would be considered some of the Wailers' finest material.

The Upsetters joined the Wailers in 1970. Aston 'Family Man' Barrett played the bass and his brother Carlton played the drums. They were unrivalled as the best rhythm section in Jamaica.

Bob and the Wailers started another label called Tuff Gong the same year and released 'Run for Cover' with a flip side of 'Sun Is Shining' as the first single. Bob, Peter, Lee Perry and Alan 'Skilly' Cole, a soccer legend and friend of Bob's, produced the Tuff Gong singles. 'Lick Samba/Samba,' 'Rat Race/Part Two,' 'Smile Jamaica Pt 1/Pt 2,' and 'Lively Up Yourself/Guava Jelly' were some of the other 45s eventually released on the label.

During the winter of 1970, Bob Marley accompanied Nash and Sims to Sweden where they were working on a movie soundtrack. He also toured with them briefly in Sweden. Upon his return to Jamaica early in 1971, the Wailers laid background vocals for some of Nash's new material which had been written by Marley.

In the meantime, the relationship between Perry and the Wailers remained tight and a hit emerged in the summer of 1971 with 'Trench Town Rock,' which was released on the English Trojan label. The song that Bob and Rita had started writing in 1967 caught on like wildfire and revitalized the Wailers' sluggish career. The Wailers continued to record with Perry on and off until 1978.

Demand renewed for Wailers' material and the band did a brisk business out of their little record shop in Kingston, dubbed the Soul Shack. The Wailers were pumping out tunes on the Tuff Gong label just to keep up with the overwhelming demand.

Towards the end of the year, the Wailers joined Nash in

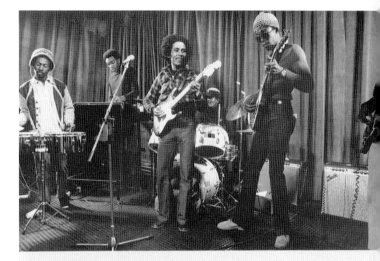

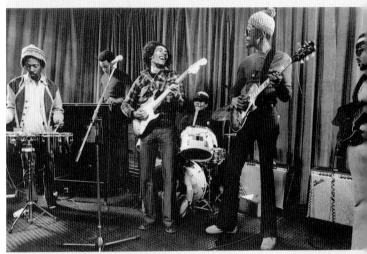

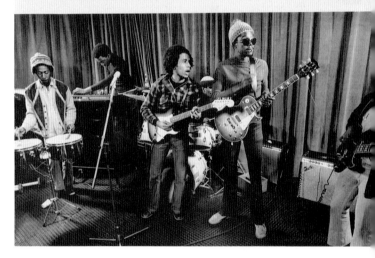

London. The album they had backed him on, *I Can See Clearly Now*, was Number One. It included four of Bob's compositions, including 'Stir It Up.'

Nash wanted the Wailers to record 'Reggae on Broadway,' a long-discussed project, to complement his album. The opportunity never materialized and Sims and Nash flew back to the States, leaving the demoralized Wailers stranded and penniless in London.

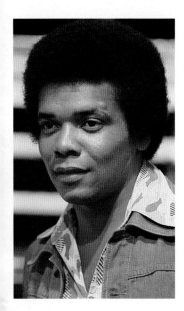

LEFT: Bob jamming and hamming it up with the Wailers in 1971.

ABOVE: American-born Johnny Nash was a recognized singer and television star from early adolescence. The Wailers served as his backup band early in their career.

RIGHT: Marley on stage in 1971, an exhausting and worrisome year for Bob and the Wailers.

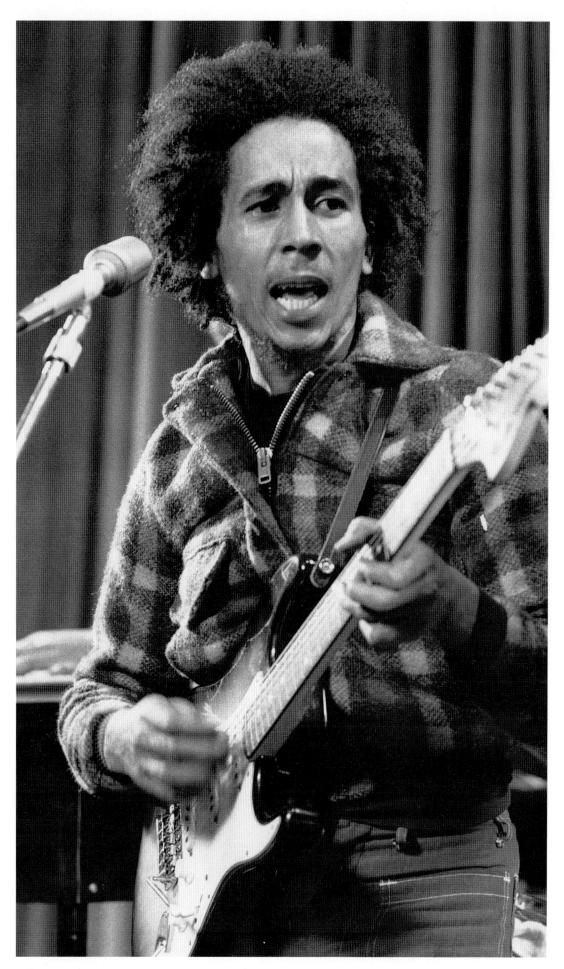

CATCH A FIRE
1972-77

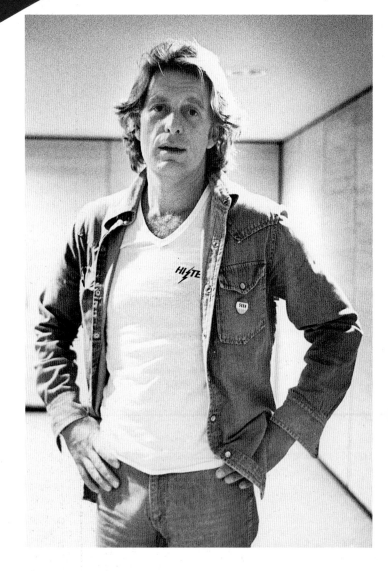

A month shy of 1972, Marley walked into Island Records' Basing Street Studios, hungry once again. He asked to see the boss, Chris Blackwell, knowing that he might be the stranded band's last chance. Blackwell, an Englishman by birth who was brought up in Jamaica, had a special bond with Rastafarians. In his youth, he was saved from certain death after a boating accident by a group of isolated Jamaican Rastas.

He was also familiar with the Jamaican recording industry. Thirteen years earlier, Blackwell made a foray into the production of Jamaican music but backed off into familiar London territory when the competition tightened in Kingston. His Island label then concentrated just on importing Jamaican music to London.

Blackwell certainly knew Bob Marley. Leslie Kong had sold him the British rights to Marley's 'One Cup of Coffee' years before. By late 1971, however, Blackwell's labels were almost

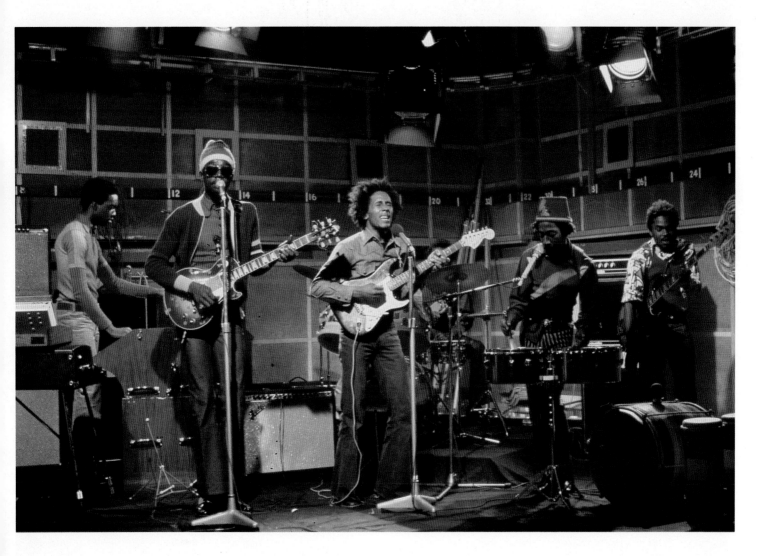

exclusively rock and roll. The only Jamaican left was Jimmy Cliff on Blackwell's Trojan label.

Apparently, Island's boss had been eyeing the Wailers for years and knew who he was dealing with when Marley walked into the room. Despite their contract with Sims, the Wailers reached an agreement with Blackwell within a few days. He gave them an £8000 advance to produce an album. The Wailers, who had only received a pittance for their recordings in the past, saw this as a sure sign of Blackwell's faith in them. It would begin a ten-year, extremely productive union between Blackwell and Marley.

Up until this point, reggae music had only been produced as singles and Blackwell wanted something new to crack the American audience. He left it up to the Wailers to create the first reggae album.

LEFT: Chris Blackwell of Island Records signed the Wailers up for their first album, *Catch a Fire* (1973).

ABOVE: The Wailers 'Stir It Up' for the crowd in 1973.

The Wailers returned to Jamaica to begin production of *Catch a Fire*. Bob used some of his share of the money to send for Rita and the children, who had been staying in Delaware. They moved to the Bull Bay Rasta settlement, six miles outside Kingston.

Production took place at three Jamaican studios: Harry J's, Dynamic Sound and Randy's. Rita and two of her friends, Judy Mowatt and Marcia Griffiths, would sometimes stop by the studios to add accompanying vocal tracks. Kingston session players helped to lay down the rhythm tracks: Tyrone Downie and Winston Wright were on keyboards, Robbie Shakespeare played bass, and Bob's 'yout,' Alvin 'Seeco' Patterson, played the hand drums.

Outside the studio, Jamaica was going through some painful rehearsals of its own. A new prime minister was about to be elected. A socialist, the PNP's Michael Manley knew the importance of the Rastafarians in this election and he aligned himself with them whenever possible.

Observing the Rastafarians' accent on the power of symbols, Manley took to carrying an African walking stick he called the 'Rod of Correction,' which he claimed was given to him by Haile

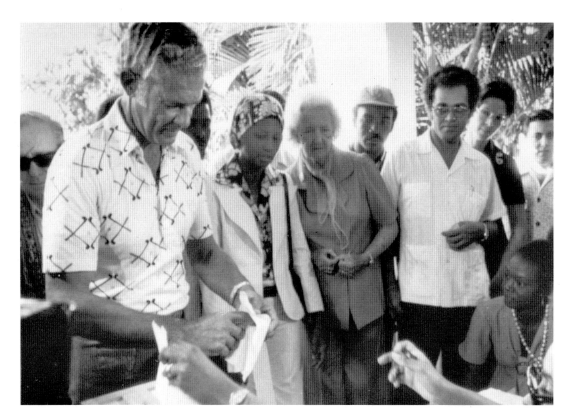

LEFT: The eccentric, politically-wise Michael Manley (left) casts his vote in the 1976 election. Manley used reggae music to curry favor with the voters.

BELOW: Following in his father's footsteps, 'Ziggy' Marley makes his first stage appearance.

Selassie. Often he cited significant Rasta bible verses and likened himself to the biblical Joshua, and his opponent to Pharaoh.

Manley was probably one of the first to realize the power of reggae music on the masses. Two songs used in the campaign by Manley, Delroy Wilson's 'Better Must Come' and the Wailers' 'Small Axe,' spoke of the intolerable living conditions of the time and hope for a better tomorrow. The Wailers didn't officially support either candidate. The ruling JLP prime minister, Hugh Shearer, banned these and other songs which were potentially detrimental to his campaign from the radio.

Manley's landmark Parliamentary majority was a clear indication that music, in particular reggae music, was the way to reach the people.

Despite the raging political turmoil outside the studios, the Wailers smoothly worked through their prepared material. By mid-year, Bob Marley was on a plane to London with the rough cuts of the album. London studio musicians filled in the blanks, and Marley and Blackwell spent the rest of the year mixing in the results.

Before the release of *Catch a Fire* in 1973, Blackwell struck a deal with Sims. He received £5000, two percent of the Wailers' next six albums and the Wailers' publishing rights. It was a sweet deal for a man who hadn't known what to do with the Wailers in the first place.

Blackwell had so much faith in the group that he hired two well-known designers, Rod Dyer and Bob Weiner, to do the

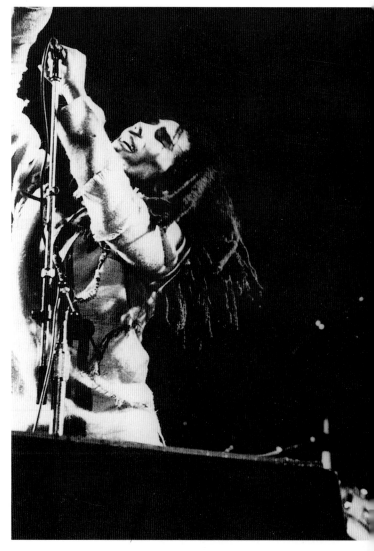

RIGHT: A still from *The Harder They Come* (1973), the film that introduced reggae music to the United States. Jimmy Cliff is pictured at left.

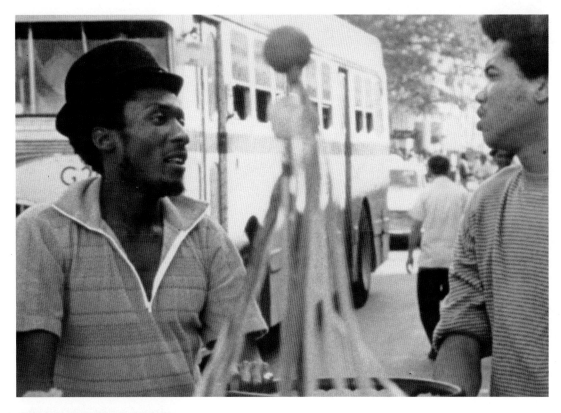

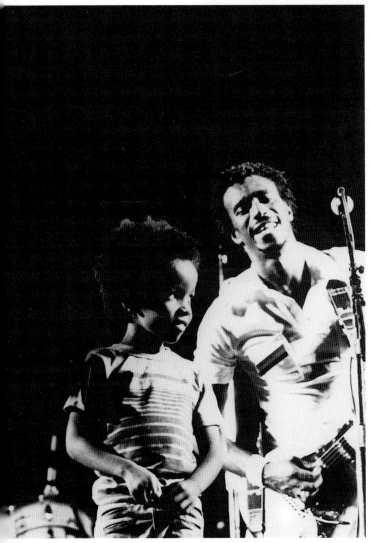

album jacket. It was an enlarged image of a Zippo lighter that opened to reveal a flame. The album became an instant collector's item for the cover alone, but it didn't hurt that the international scene was ripe for the likes of 'Concrete Jungle' and 'Stir It Up.'

The Wailers' first Island album was a great success in Britain, but the American audience was less familiar with reggae music. American critics, however, embraced the rebel lyrics and the hip-shaking beat, and the album sold 14,000 copies in the United States in the first year, despite very little promotion by American distributors.

Another of Blackwell's interests, a small investment in the film *The Harder They Come*, would pay off for him in more ways than one that year. Released in the States in 1973, the movie sparked an interest in reggae music. Blackwell's subsequent release of the soundtrack helped start the American careers of Toots & the Maytals, Third World and the Heptones. The Wailers' album also fed the new American hunger and it sold briskly.

The Wailers were booked by Island for a spring tour of England and a summer and fall tour of the States. They also began work on their second Island album, as specified by their contract with Blackwell.

The Wailers now numbered six, including a fresh new keyboard player named Earl 'Wire' Lindo. Once in London, it didn't take the Wailers long to find out that their next album had been released. However, it wasn't the album they had been working on in Jamaica.

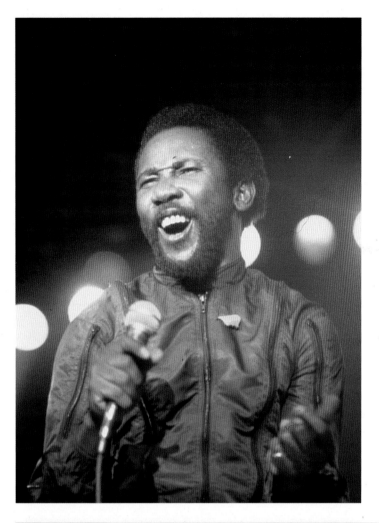

African Herbsman was released in the spring of 1973 on the Trojan label. Trojan, which had once belonged to Blackwell, now belonged to his estranged partner Lee Goptal. Noting the Wailers' rising popularity, Lee 'Scratch' Perry sold the rights to some of the Wailers' earlier work to Goptal. It was then compiled into an album. Included on the album were 'Small Axe,' 'Trench Town Rock,' 'Duppy Conquerer,' and 'Lively Up Yourself.' The release coincided with the beginning of the English tour, and the Wailers played to packed arenas.

At the end of May, they appeared on the BBC's 'Old Grey Whistle Test' and played 'Concrete Jungle' and 'Stop that Train,' both from *Catch a Fire*. The next week they gave a concert which was radio broadcast from the BBC's Paris Theatre. Despite tensions within the band, they set the audience on fire with their magical blend of rebellion and sexually-charged rhythms.

After a ninety-day whirlwind tour, they returned to Jamaica and Bunny said he would never tour outside of Jamaica again. He never did.

In July, the American leg of the tour began in New England. Joe Higgs replaced Bunny and the band started by playing to an all-white, jubilant crowd at Paul's Mall in Boston. The band at this point consisted of Higgs, Marley, Tosh, Wire and the Barrett brothers. Then they headed south for Max's Kansas City in New York City where they opened for Bruce Springsteen.

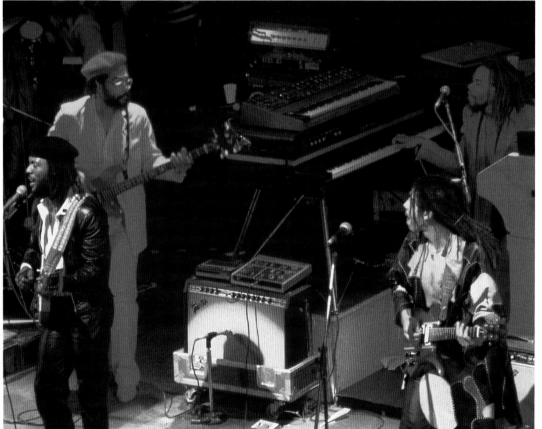

TOP LEFT: Toots and the Maytals became popular in the United States at the same time as the Wailers. Shown here is Toots Hibbert.

LEFT: Still playing to packed US audiences today, Third World came from humble beginnings.

TOP RIGHT: Marley takes a rest before a show in Berlin.

RIGHT: Bob practices a new type of soccer header in Stockholm, Sweden.

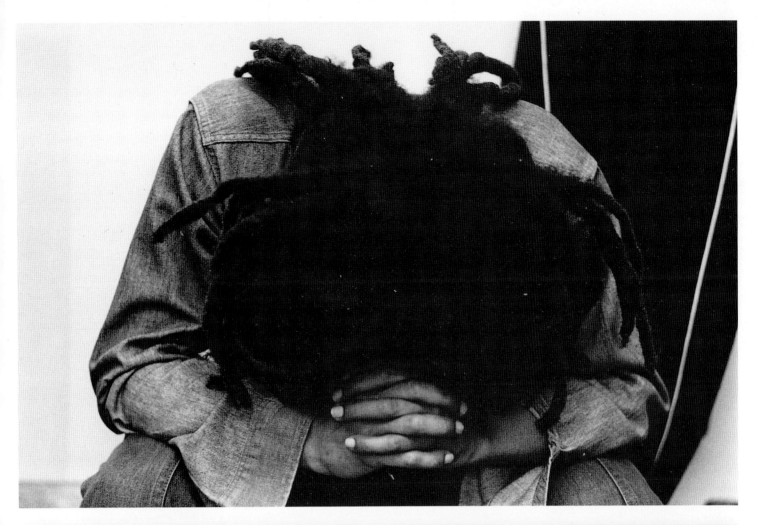

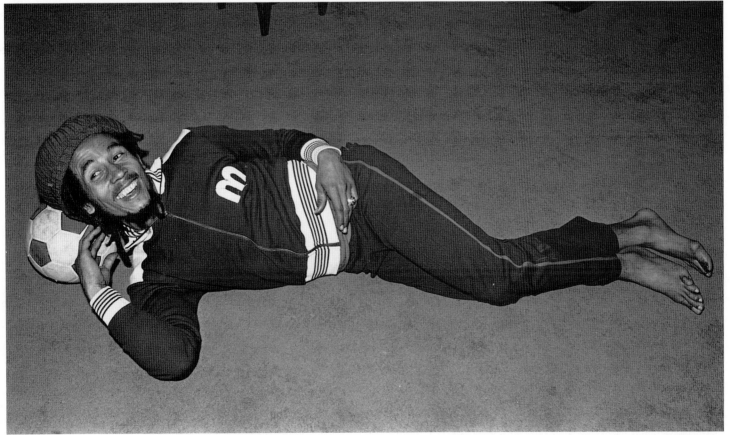

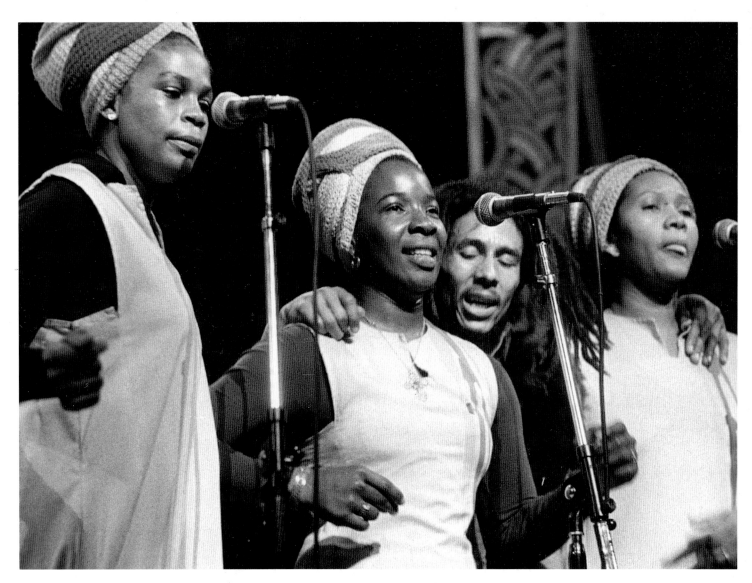

Bob's mother, her husband and their children came up to see the band's three New York City sets. Afterwards, at a party in Brooklyn, everyone met Rita's father who was visiting from Sweden. It was a jubilant, though hectic time.

The Wailers' first 'disappointment' came in October when they played with Sly and the Family Stone in Las Vegas. After four shows they were fired because they were showing up the headliners.

Upon their return to Jamaica, the Wailers lived at Island House at 56 Hope Road, Kingston, which was owned by Blackwell. The Wailers had moved uptown, much to the dismay of their all-white, upper class neighbors. Island House became a bustling Rasta commune of sorts. Surrounded by the lush, tropical vegetation, the men would play soccer on the grounds and work out new tunes on their guitars on the porch.

The band's second album, *Burnin'*, was released in October 1973. The album was a response to what they believed was Michael Manley's false-prophet election of 1972. It included 'Get

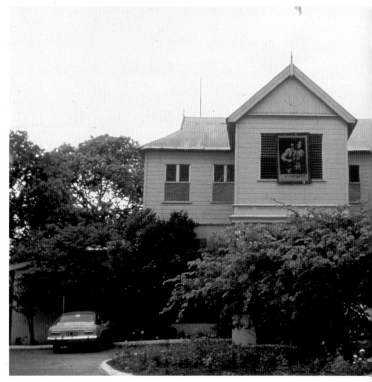

LEFT: Bob rocks with the I-Threes at the Rainbow Theatre in London in 1977. Rita is pictured in the middle.

RIGHT: An exuberant Bob Marley in London, 1975.

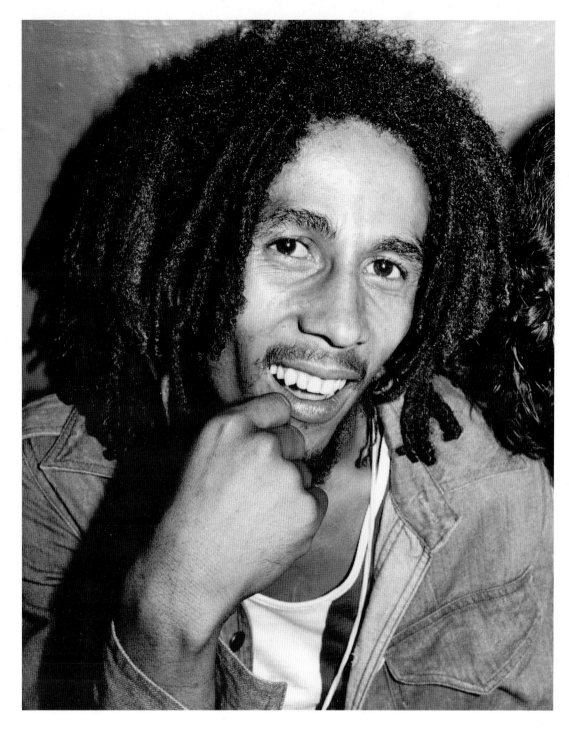

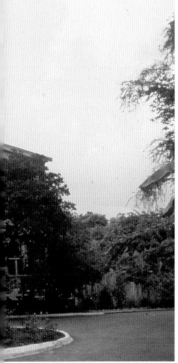

LEFT: Moving uptown: 56 Hope Road in Kingston, the playground of the Rasta musicians from the slums.

Up, Stand Up,' 'I Shot the Sheriff,' 'Burnin' and Lootin',' a new version of 'Duppy Conquerer,' and 'Small Axe.' It was a revolutionary album that encouraged people to recognize their situation and do something to improve it.

It was also a particularly vicious indictment of Manley, who they felt had abandoned them. They let him know that they wouldn't be fooled by him again. Since his installment as prime minister, which had been largely due to Rasta support, he had done little to improve the conditions of the Rasta man. Max Romeo, a well-known Rasta singer, also came out with an indictment of Manley with 'No Joshua No.'

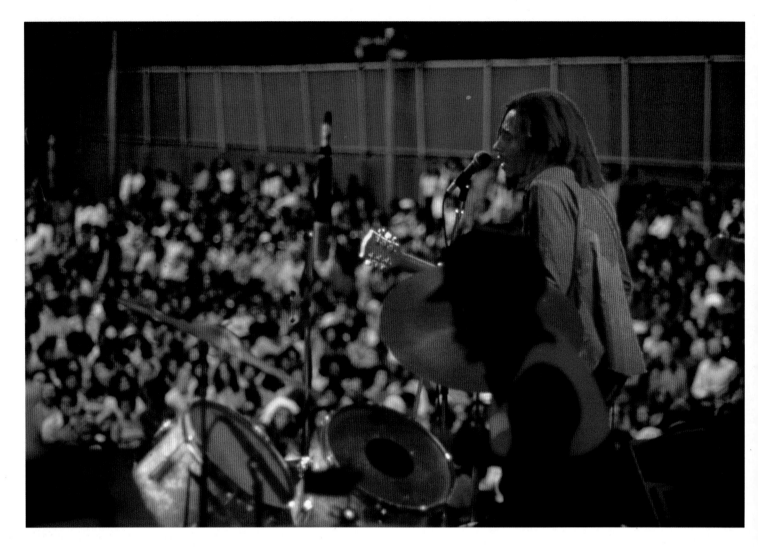

Manley declared a democratic socialist government which allowed free speech and press for all. When the *Burnin'* album was released, prior to Manley's declaration, it included printed lyrics and the Wailers had already established themselves as spokespeople for the Rastafarian movement. It also generated a great deal of publicity in the States, where they were still considered somewhat of an oddity.

In August 1974 Eric Clapton released *461 Ocean Boulevard*, which included a cover version of 'I Shot the Sheriff.' It was a US and Jamaican pop chart sensation. Surprisingly, Barbra Streisand also did a cover of a Bob Marley and the Wailers song: the version of 'Guava Jelly' appeared on her *Butterfly* album.

The Wailers were on the edge of American success. In order to help ensure the success of the group in the States, Blackwell introduced them to Al Anderson, a black American rock guitarist, who became a welcome addition to the group.

Later in the year, Bob and Blackwell had a falling out, delaying the release of *Natty Dread*, originally titled *Knotty Dread*. The band was also kicked out of 56 Hope Road. The feud was soon resolved, but clearly Blackwell was pressuring Bob.

At the beginning of 1975, the original Wailers, Bunny, Bob and Peter, officially parted ways. Bunny and Peter had sensed that Blackwell's agenda for the group did not include them. Tosh had approached Blackwell earlier to see if he would produce a solo album for him. When Blackwell responded that he believed it would compromise the integrity of the Wailers, Peter was furious. Bunny's unwillingness to tour made his departure a natural step. One thing led to another and they agreed a break would be good for all of them.

The new 'Bob Marley and the Wailers' played with the Jackson Five at a concert in Kingston, Jamaica. They were backed by the I-Threes: Rita Marley, Judy Mowatt and Marcia Griffiths.

TOP: By 1975 every Wailers show was packed with a multitude of joyful, adoring fans.

RIGHT: The confident, enlightened Natty Dread.

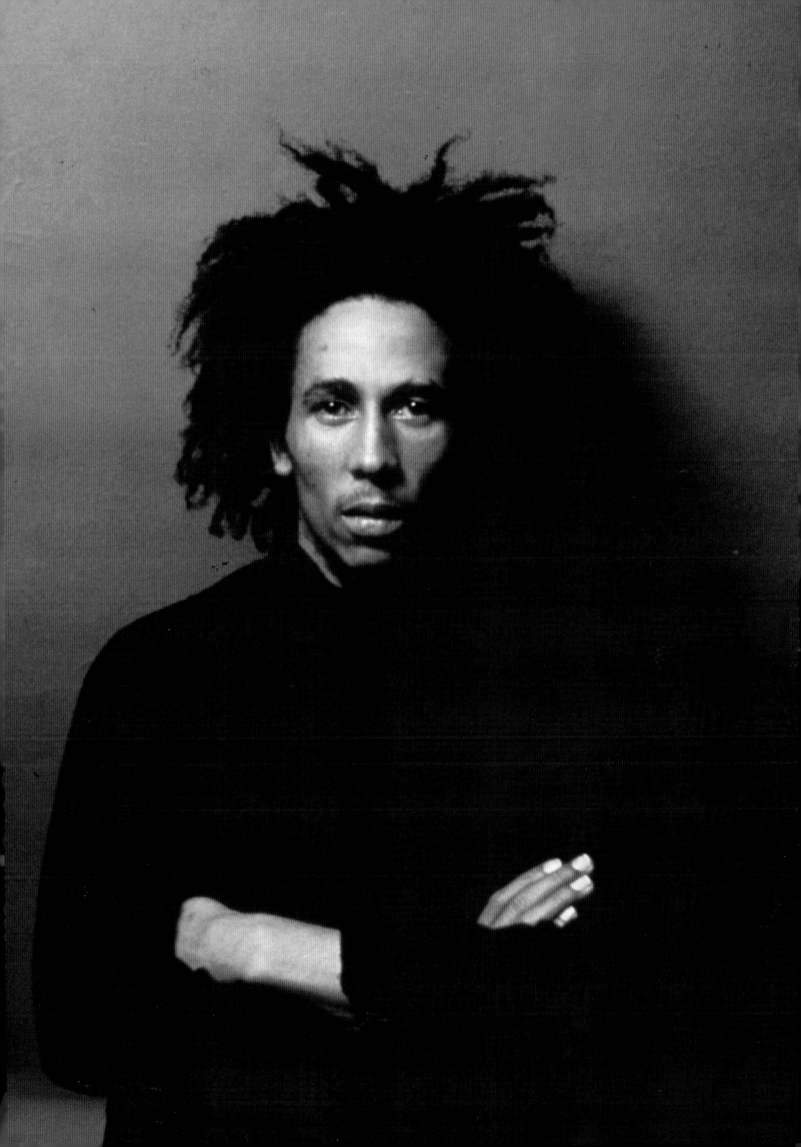

The new ensemble began touring the States in June 1975 to promote *Natty Dread*, which had finally been released by Island in late 1974. They played many of the tunes from the new album, including 'Lively Up Yourself,' which featured Al Anderson prominently on guitar, 'No Woman No Cry,' 'Them Belly Full, But We Hungry,' 'Rebel Music,' and 'Revolution.' It was considered a strongly militant album and appealed to young revolution-minded audiences around the world.

The Diplomat Hotel in Hollywood, Florida was the first stop on the tour. As usual, the musicians played against the backdrop of Rasta colors, the symbol of the Lion of Judah, and a portrait of Haile Selassie I. Next came Canada, Philadelphia, Boston, New York's Central Park, Cleveland, Detroit, and Chicago. They played to ecstatic crowds in California. San Francisco's Boarding House and Los Angeles' Roxy appearances were noted as being particularly explosive. Every musician in America had his eye on Bob Marley and the evolution of reggae music.

The tour then moved to Europe, and in London on 18 July 1975 the Wailers recorded their first all-live LP, *Live! at the Lyceum*. It was released as soon as possible and would later read like a greatest hits album. It included the smash favorites 'Trench Town Rock,' 'Burnin' and Lootin',' 'No Woman No Cry,' 'I Shot the Sheriff,' and 'Get Up, Stand Up.' Marley was developing a cult-like following, and the Lyceum recording demonstrates their fervent devotion to the Rasta prophet. The album sold heavily wherever the band toured in Europe and the States. The day after the concert a picture of Bob playing soccer appeared in the British magazine *New Music Express*.

On 27 August 1975, Haile Selassie I died. Opponents of the Rastafarian movement claimed their God was dead and hadn't redeemed them after all. Selassie had also become a reviled figure in his native Ethiopia, where he was dethroned and imprisoned some years before his death. He was buried in an unmarked grave.

In response to these accusations, Bob interrupted the recording of a new album to record 'Jah Live' in September. It appeared as a message to Marley's brethren that God can't be killed, and that Selassie's spirit was still alive and well. The message was as mysterious to non-believers as the religion was itself.

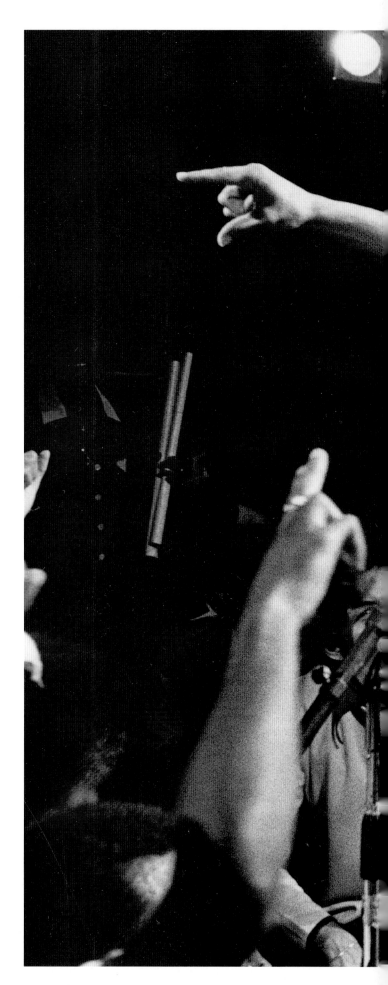

RIGHT: **Pointing towards revolution: Live at the Lyceum, London, 1975.**

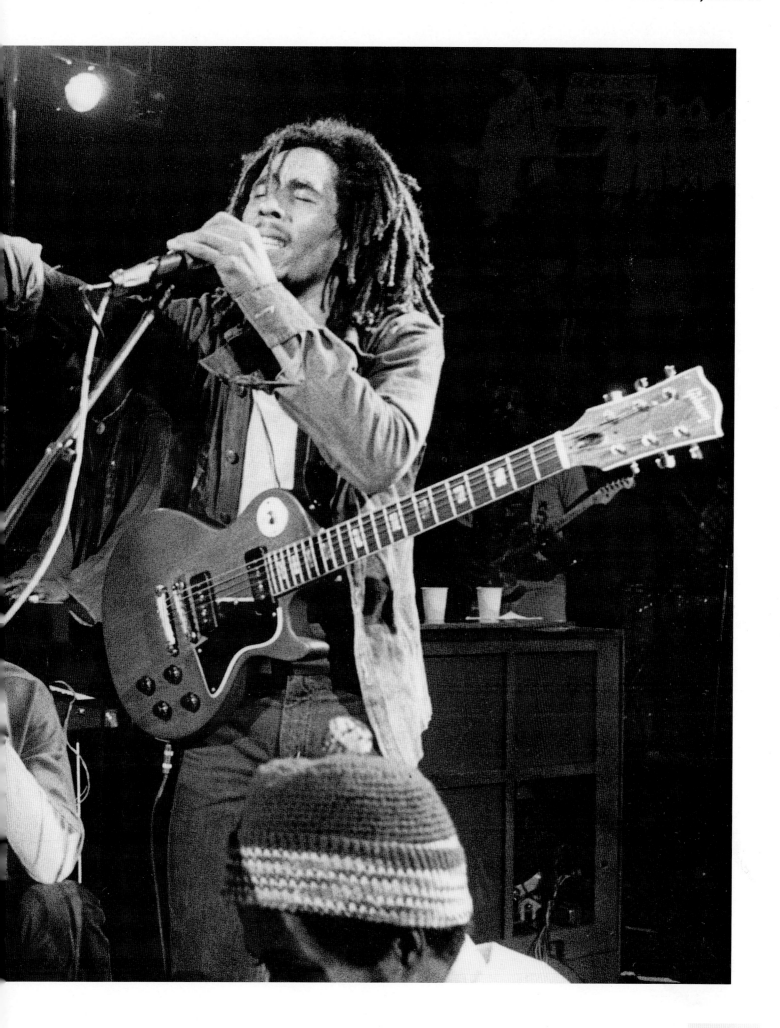

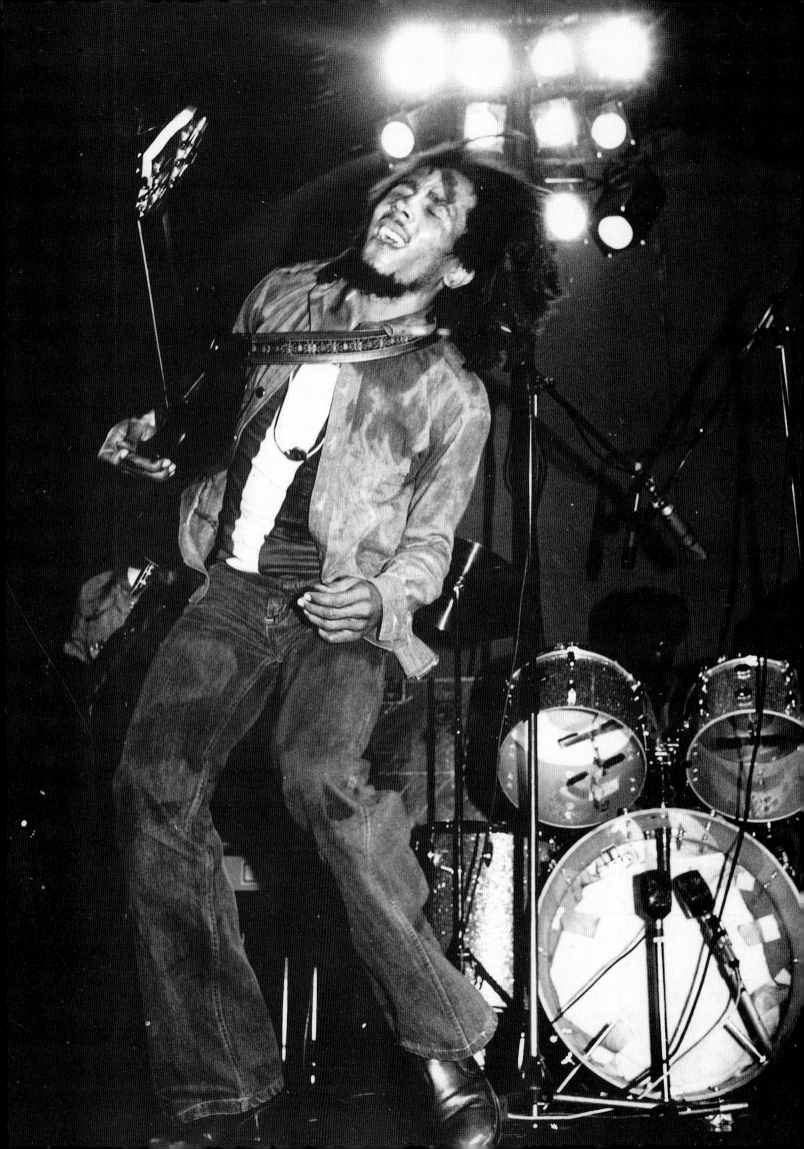

On 11 September, two reggae articles appeared in *Rolling Stone* magazine. One was entitled 'Marley, the Maytals and the Reggae Armageddon,' the other 'An Herbal Meditation with Bob Marley.' The articles attempted to explain the Caribbean movement so misunderstood by American audiences and to define reggae music. The publicity caused Marley's popularity to skyrocket.

In November, the three original Wailers rejoined to play a benefit concert in Kingston. They played with Stevie Wonder, the top black recording artist at the time, to benefit the Jamaican Institute for the Blind. They performed for a feverish audience until four in the morning.

In early 1976, the reggae craze hit the US and Marleymania was official. Photographs and articles about Bob appeared in nearly every publication, including the *New York Times*. The Wailers were proclaimed 'Band of the Year' in the 12 February issue of *Rolling Stone*.

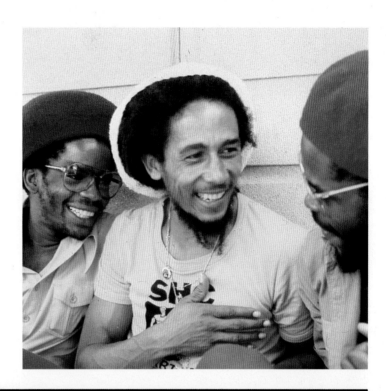

LEFT: Marley delivers the fire under the hot lights of the Lyceum in London, 1975.

TOP RIGHT: Members of the band share a jovial moment at Hope Road in 1975.

RIGHT: A bird's eye view of a 1976 Wailers performance.

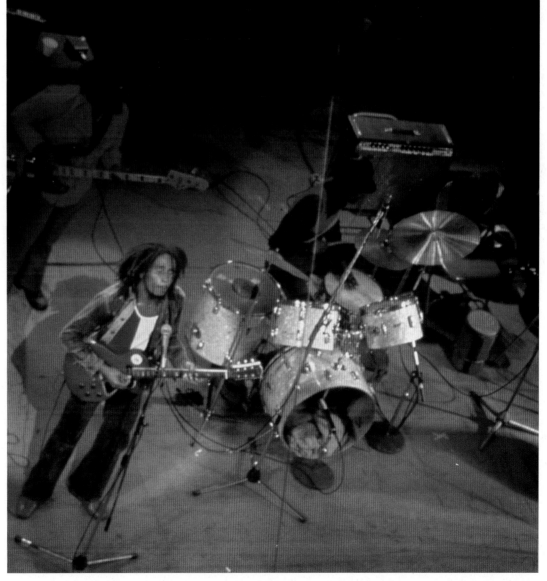

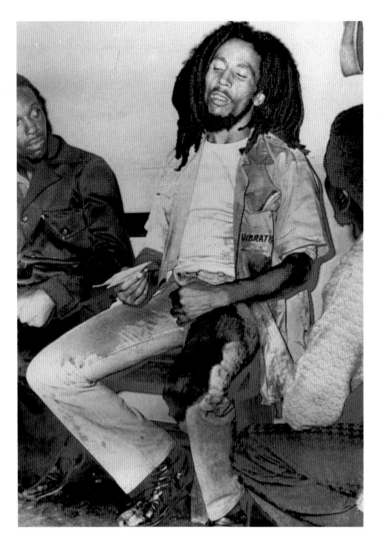

To help bring peace back to the troubled land, Bob and the Wailers agreed to do a free concert in Kingston's National Heroes Park on 5 December 1976. The government announced that elections would be held a few weeks after the concert. Manley hoped that the timing of the concert would make it look like the Wailers were endorsing him for re-election, although they supported neither candidate.

Strange things began happening to the Hope Road gang, and Bob was receiving anonymous death threats for his involvement in the concert. On the evening of 3 December 1976, the group was on a quick break from concert rehearsals. Bob walked to the kitchen with Don Kinsey for some grapefruit. They were soon joined by Wailers promoter Don Taylor. Shots rang out and the windows shattered. Rita Marley was struck by one of the six gunmen's bullets as she was attempting to shepherd the children to safety.

Another gunman entered the kitchen and shot at Marley and Taylor. Taylor took five bullets, inadvertently saving Bob's life. Bob was grazed in the ribs by a bullet that then passed through his arm.

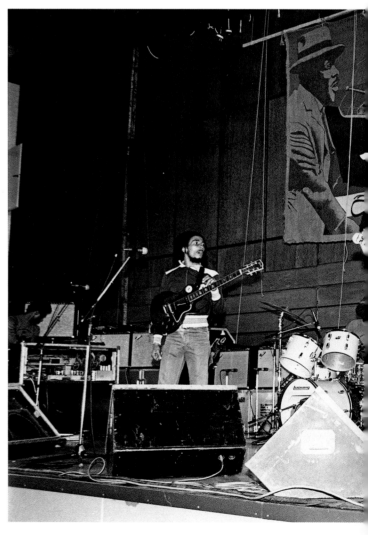

During that time, Al Anderson left the Wailers to play with Tosh and was replaced by Earl 'Chinna' Smith, of Soul Syndicate fame, and the blues guitarist Don Kinsey.

In May, *Rastaman Vibration*, the fifth Blackwell-Marley collaboration, was released in the United States. It was rather disappointing to diehard fans who craved the hard-edged rebellion music. However, his media notoriety created a new group of fans who made the album Marley's biggest seller to date. 'Rat Race' and 'Johnny Was' expressed Bob's bitterness toward upcoming elections in Jamaica. 'War' was a derivation of an anti-racism speech given by Haile Selassie I in 1968.

In June, the Wailers toured the US again to support the album. At the end of the show at the Tower Theatre, Philadelphia, nine-year-old Ziggy joined his father on stage for a little song and dance.

Jamaica was under martial law following a spring and early summer of violence. Pre-election violence had become a Jamaican tradition but seemed to be fueled by outside forces this time. Guns were more easily accessible and food supplies were dwindling.

FAR LEFT: **Bob Marley waits at the University Hospital in Kingston after being shot by gunmen who invaded his home on 3 December 1976.**

BELOW: **The band tunes up in Frankfurt, Germany, on 2 April 1977 in front of a banner honoring Marcus Garvey.**

RIGHT: **An older-looking Bob tunes up with Family Man in Berlin, 1977.**

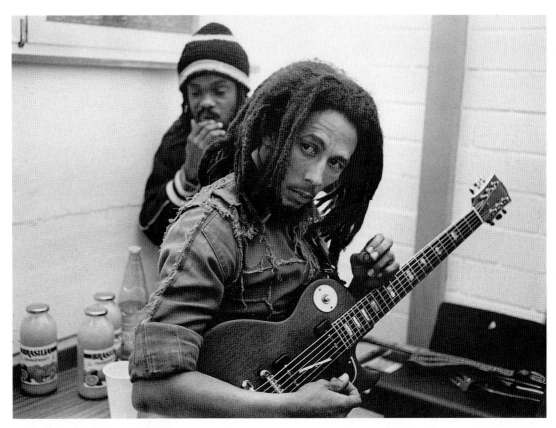

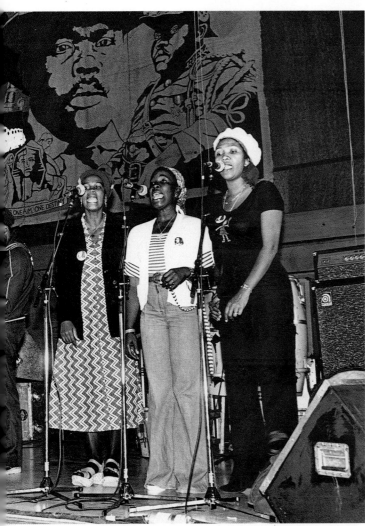

As quickly as they had arrived, the gunmen disappeared, leaving four people injured, two critically. Everyone fully recovered, but Bob was whisked into hiding by Manley and the PNP until the concert.

The 'Smile Jamaica' concert went ahead as planned, with the Marleys appearing in bandages. Bob started his 90-minute set with 'War.' The opportunistic Manley stood on top of a van, in full view of any gunmen, for the rest of the show.

Bob was shaken by the shooting, and despite the success of the concert he flew out of Jamaica the next morning and into exile. On 16 December, Manley defeated his JLP opponent Edward Seaga, capturing a huge majority in the Jamaican House of Representatives.

The Wailers spent most of 1977 in London recording their new, aptly titled *Exodus* album. A new guitarist, Junior Marvin, was brought in for the sessions. 'Natural Mystic,' 'Jamming,' 'Exodus,' 'Three Little Birds,' and 'One Love/People Get Ready' were among the Wailers' offerings that year.

The reggae group Culture had a smash hit that year called 'Two Sevens Clash,' based on the Rasta belief that 1977 would be a significant year for the brethren. Some even thought that 7 July 1977 would mark the end of the world. That year, Bob Marley had a private audience with Haile Selassie's grandson, who was also exiled in London. It was Crown Prince Asfa Wossan who gave Marley the coveted Lion of Judah ring.

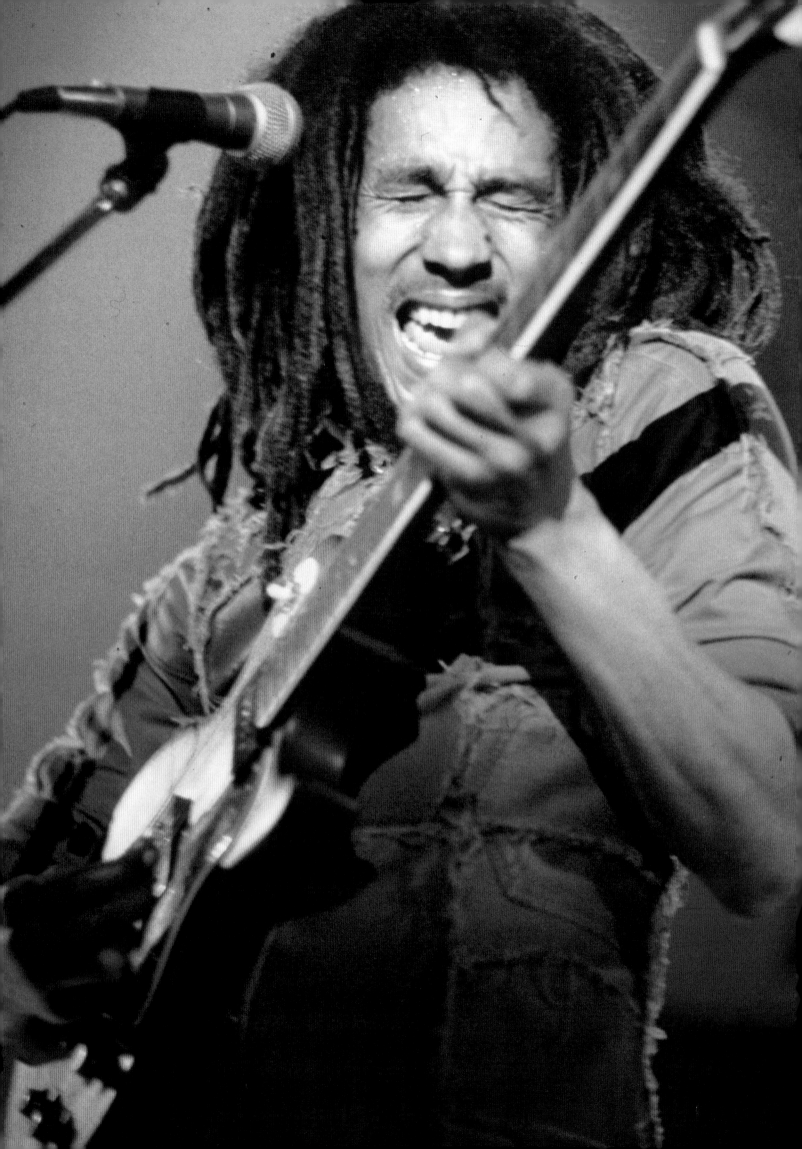

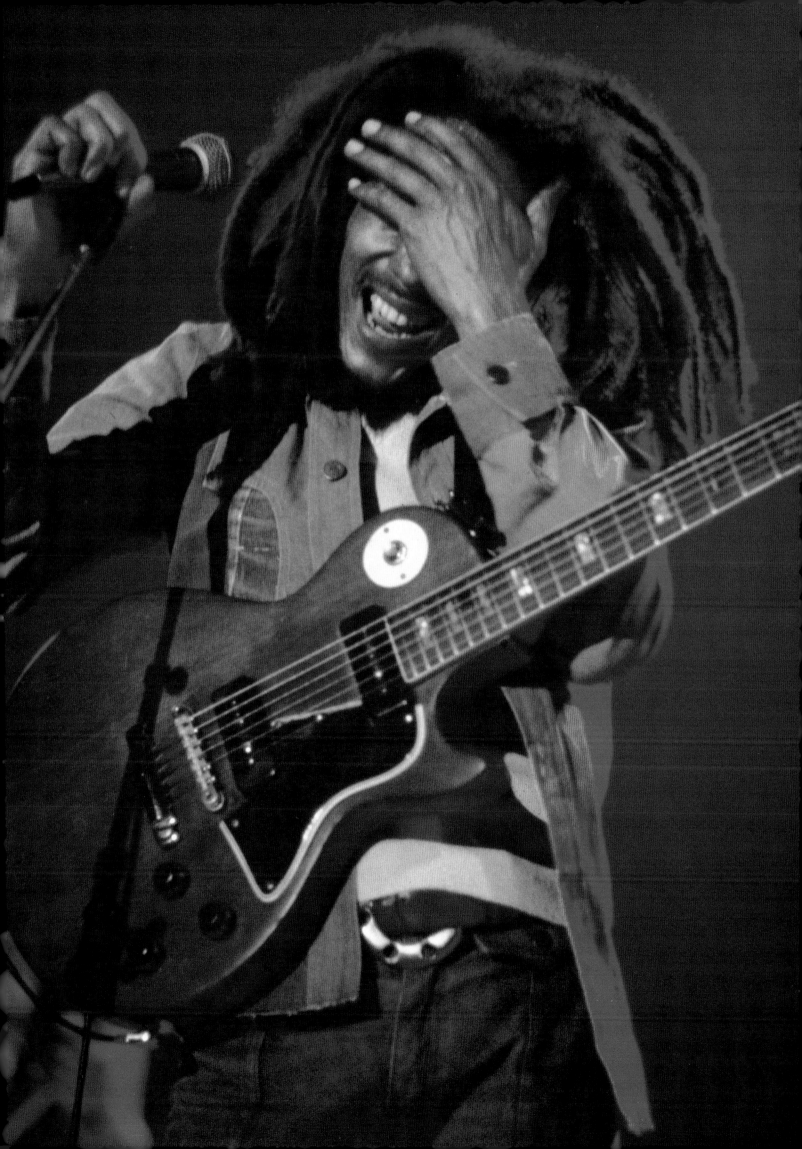

During the May 1977 tour of Europe, Bob was playing soccer with the Wailers and some French journalists when he injured his foot. The same toe had been injured years before and had taken some time to heal. This time it didn't heal at all, and Bob reluctantly went to a doctor a month later in England. The doctor told him he had cancer and that part of the toe would have to be amputated.

Bob refused, due to his Rasta beliefs, and decided that the only alternative was to rest. The rest of the Exodus tour was cancelled on 20 July.

PREVIOUS PAGES AND THESE PAGES:
Scenes from the 1977 Exodus tour in Europe.

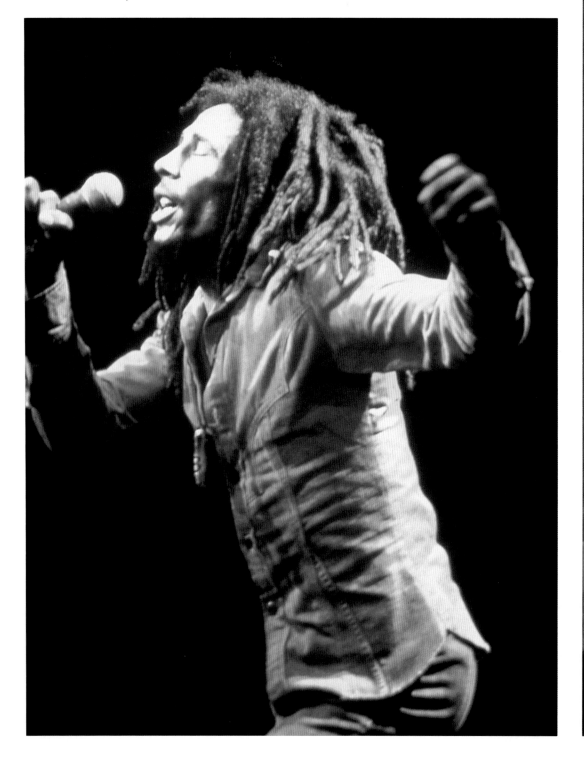

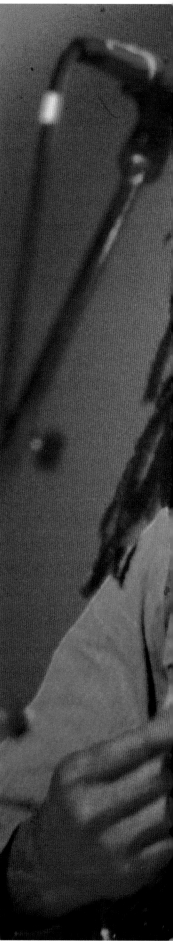

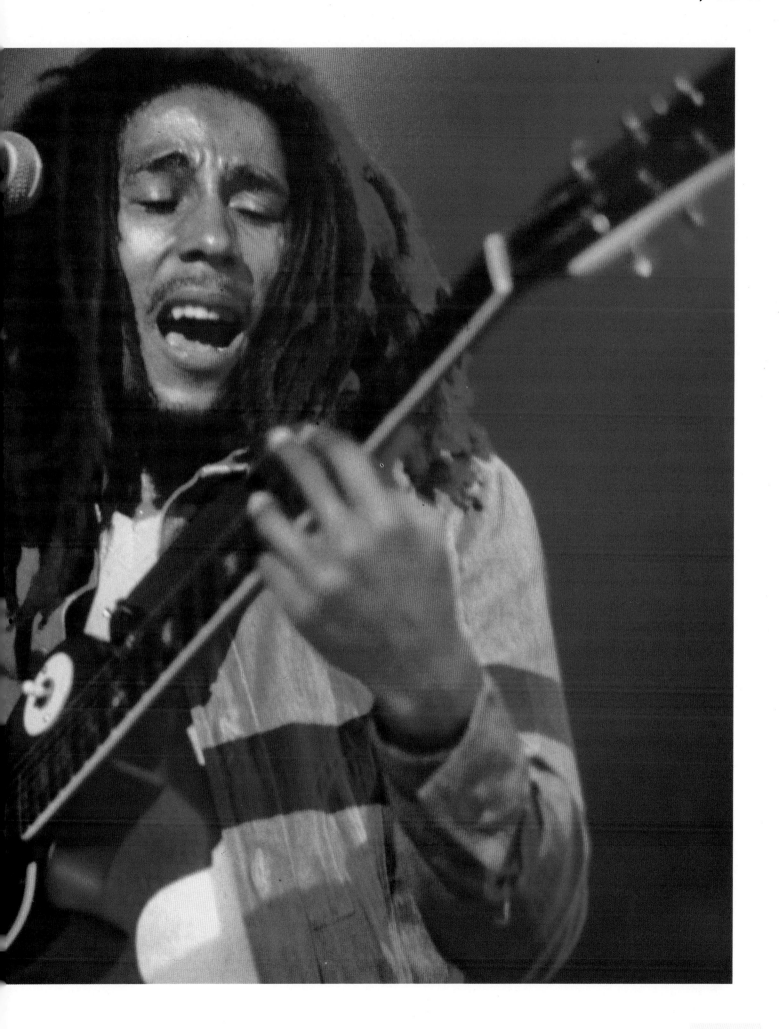

BUFFALO SOLDIER
1978-81

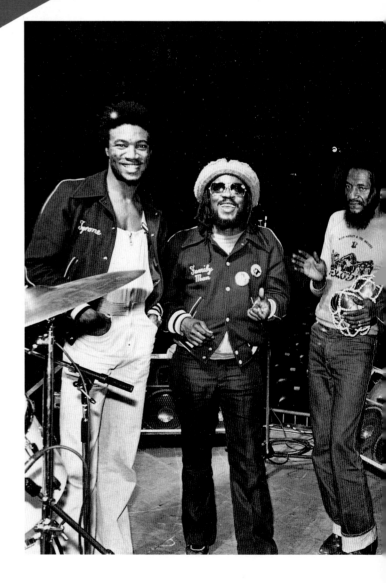

Despite the cancelled tour, *Exodus* sold well in the States. However, the US was still uncharted territory for reggae musicians in 1978 and Bob and the Wailers had to carve a niche for themselves in the already crowded world of rock and roll. They were fighting a valiant battle on the American music frontier against such greats as the Rolling Stones, Bob Dylan, and Stevie Wonder.

In May of that year, Bob recorded a song called 'Buffalo Soldier,' written by Jamaican producer King Sporty. The song was recorded in Miami and compared Jamaican Rastafarians, or 'dreadlock Rastas,' to the black American soldiers during the US Civil War. 'Buffalo Soldier' is a very revealing glimpse of Marley during this period in his life.

Bob and his family had recently survived an attack on their lives and were alienated from their homeland. Similarly, the

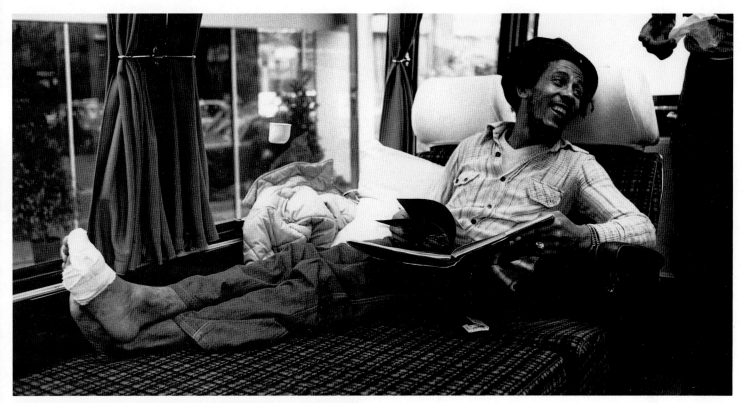

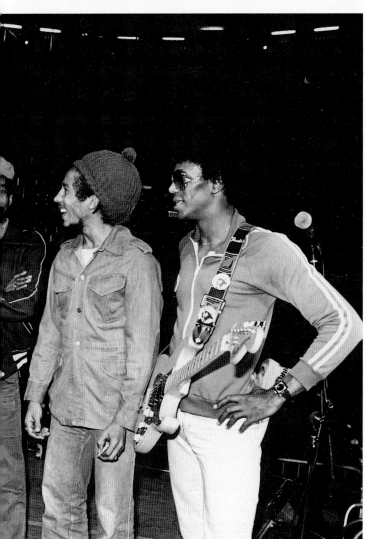

'Buffalo Soldiers' were stolen from Africa against their wills and were fighting a battle in a foreign land. The soldiers changed the face of American soldiering forever, just as Marley changed the music scene forever. Both were part of the political landscape in spite of their difficulties in addressing it.

Despite his physical removal from the historically violent political scene, Bob was still a part of it, spiritually. Two of his friends, Claudie 'Jack' Massop, a big man in the JLP, and Bucky Marshall, a PNP underling, were sharing a jail cell back in Kingston. They discussed the unsettling tensions among the people that year. The streets of Jamaica were sweltering in the heat of tribal warfare, thanks in part to the gun problem.

LEFT: **The Wailers onstage before the Gothenberg, Sweden, show.**

TOP: **Bob rests on the Wailers' tour bus in Europe after injuring his toe in 1977.**

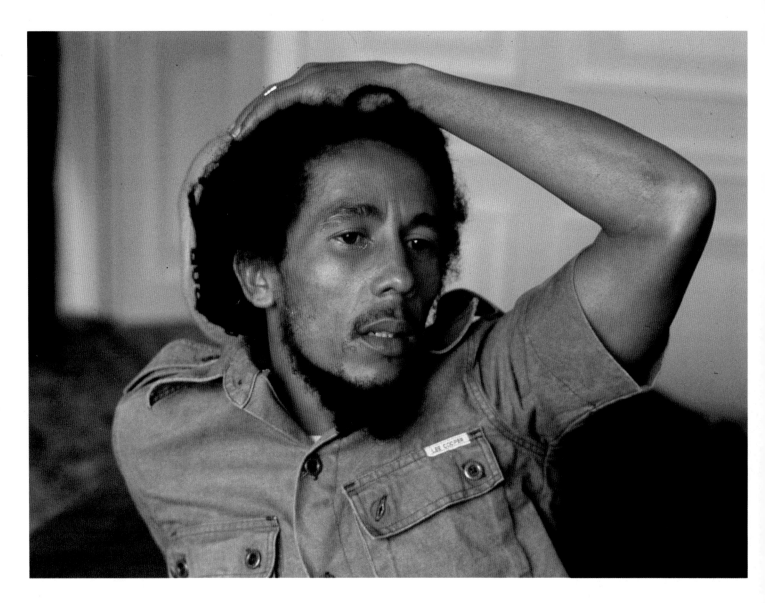

Gun-wielding Jamaicans were turning against each other in droves. Women and children were being raped in horrifying numbers and men were dying on the streets like flies. People were emigrating as quickly as they could scrape up the airfare.

Massop and Marshall realized that while their ideologies were different, neither one of them was benefitting from a civil war. The two arranged a truce between their political factions. To cement the deal, they concocted a national concert called the One Love Peace Concert, scheduled for 22 April 1978. Bob would be invited to headline.

Bob had not been back to Jamaica since his exodus after the shooting. In his absence, 'Bob Marley and the Wailers' records did not sell well in Jamaica. Many people believed he had sold out to the international scene or to the PNP. However, Massop and Marshall realized his return would send a strong signal to the island. If Marley was willing to return to a country everyone was leaving, especially in light of what happened to him in 1976, there must be some hope left.

They needed an impartial messenger to deliver the request to Marley, who was now living in Florida with his mother, Rita and their children. Massop and Marshall contacted the Twelve Tribes of Israel, a Rastafarian sect to which Marley belonged. Prophet Gad (Vernon Carrington), the leader of the tribe, agreed to sponsor the peace movement and act as a go-between.

TOP: **Bob answers questions during a 1978 interview.**

RIGHT: **Bob in exile, before being wooed to return to Jamaica for the One Love Peace Concert in 1978.**

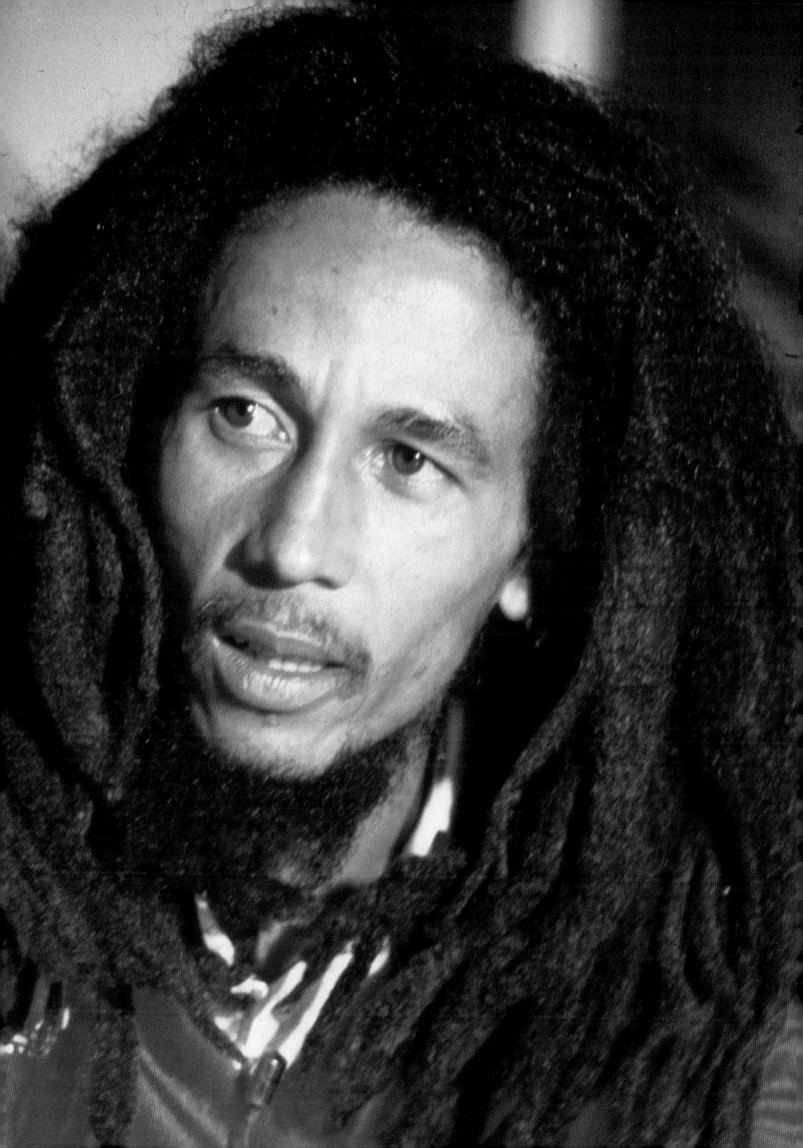

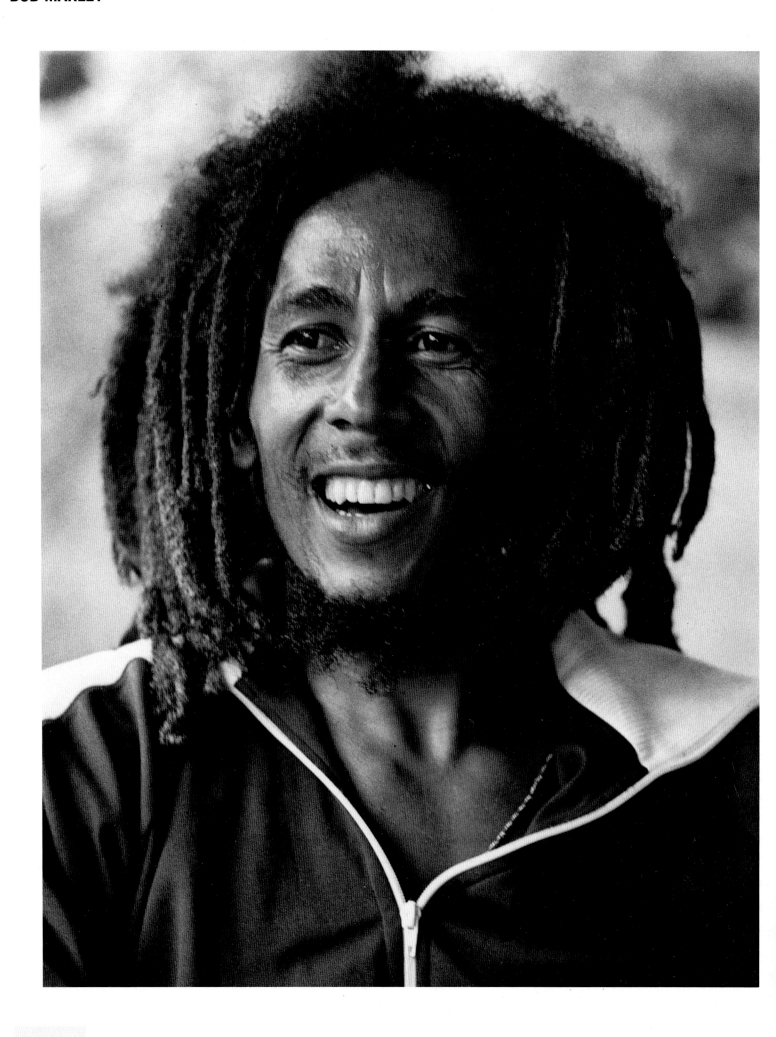

LEFT: **The photo of Bob that was used on the *Kaya* album cover.**

RIGHT: **The I-Threes: left to right, Judy Mowatt, Rita Marley, Marcia Griffiths.**

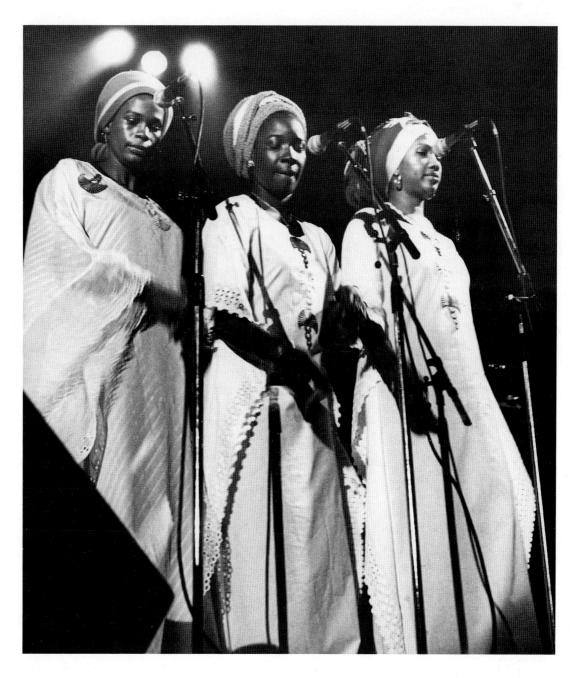

Wisely skeptical of the ensuing proposition, Marley requested a meeting with Massop on neutral London soil. In early February, Marley demanded his unconditional safe passage and that of his family and band, if they should decide to return. Apparently, Massop confirmed the political nature of the shooting during their initial meeting, but assured Marley that all was well for his return. Later, a representative of the PNP was sent to join the talks.

Though hesitant at first, Marley eventually felt the concert would serve as an essential salve to the burning wound that Jamaica had become. The 23rd of February marked the official announcement of the ghetto truce and subsequent concert.

Within two weeks, Bob returned to Hope Road where a delegation greeted him joyfully. The Wailers re-formed and started rehearsing for the upcoming concert, which would begin a world tour to promote *Kaya*, another Island release. A week after the album's release in Britain, it hit Number Four on the charts. Ironically, *Kaya* was a far cry from Bob's defiant 'Get Up, Stand Up'-type protest songs. It was essentially a collection of love songs.

During March interviews in New York, Marley reiterated his dedication to the Jamaican poor and his willingness and intention to fight for better conditions. He hadn't given up; his angle had just changed slightly. It was clear that hard-edged protest wasn't working in the slum's streets, so maybe a little love and forgiveness would.

Fervent, security-clogged rehearsals continued at Hope Road. Massop was a visible figure in the compound to personally ensure Bob's safety.

In the unfortunate Jamaican tradition, violence erupted in West Kingston on 17 April, just days before the concert. It had been clear from the start that much of the proceeds from the concert were going towards construction of better housing and sanitary facilities in the ghettos. A peaceful protest of these poor conditions ended with three dead. Apparently, government security forces, acting of their own accord, gunned down the protesters.

Following the shooting, a staunch warning was issued by the security minister, Dudley Thompson. He made it clear that any retaliatory acts for the shootings would result in immediate death for the criminal. Clearly, there was tension in the air.

Despite the violence, throngs of people crowded the streets of Kingston to get tickets to the concert at the National Stadium. The three sections of the stadium were renamed 'Love,' 'Peace' and 'Togetherness' for the occasion.

Besides Marley and the Wailers, the six hour show starred Peter Tosh, Culture, Big Youth, The Mighty Diamonds, Dennis Brown, and Jacob Miller and Inner Circle. Miller sang his specially written 'The Peace Treaty Special.' Nearly every top performer in

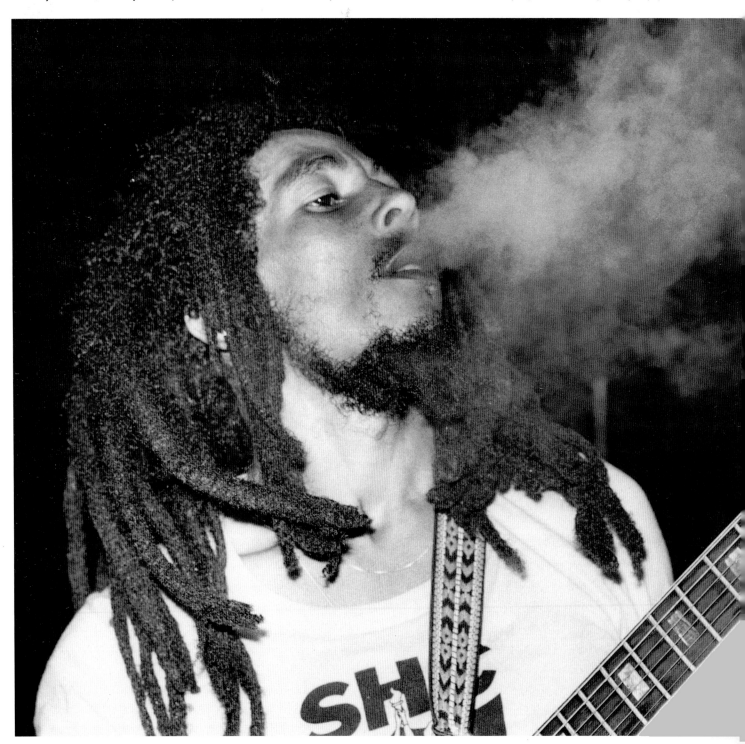

BELOW: Bob exhales a cloud of smoke during a sound check before the One Love Peace Concert in Kingston, Jamaica, on 22 April 1978.

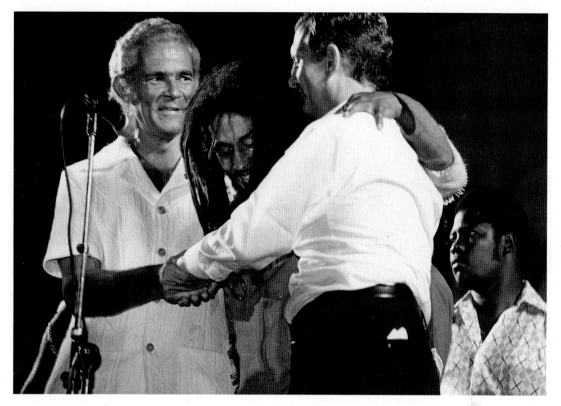

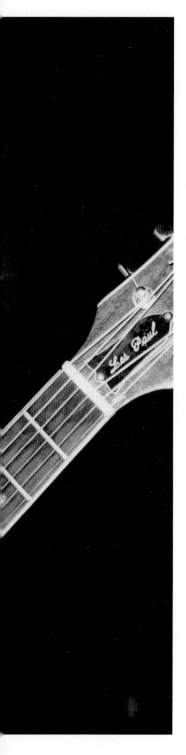

ABOVE: Marley unites stiff-handed rival politicians Michael Manley and Edward Seaga in a powerful embrace during the One Love Peace Concert.

Jamaica appeared onstage that night pleading for the truce to continue and urging the youths to stop killing each other. However, Bunny Wailer, skeptical of the truce's sincerity, boycotted the show and refused to play.

Following Peter Tosh's set, which included a strong reprimand of Seaga and Manley for their false promises, the Wailers sauntered onstage. The crowd went wild.

Most of the songs were from the *Exodus* album, but the Wailers set the stage by starting with 'Trench Town Rock.' Its images were clearly an indictment of the current conditions. Later, Marley looked skyward and warned that 'the Lion of Judah will break every chain and give us victory again and again.'

Soon afterwards, he coaxed arch-enemies Seaga and Manley onstage. The crowd watched in utter disbelief as Marley joined their hands together over his head. It was an incredible, symbolic moment for Jamaica. Marley tied up the concert appropriately with its namesake, 'One Love.'

For the next month, Bob rehearsed the Wailers and the I-Threes exhaustively for the Kaya tour. Tyrone Downie and Earl 'Wire' Lindo were on keyboards, Junior Marvin and Al Anderson (who had rejoined the band) on guitar, the Barrett brothers and Alvin 'Seeco' Patterson rounded out the rhythm section and the I-Threes provided backup vocals.

Three singles from the new album were released: Island put out 'Satisfy My Soul' and 'Is This Love,' and Tuff Gong followed suit with 'Blackman Redemption.'

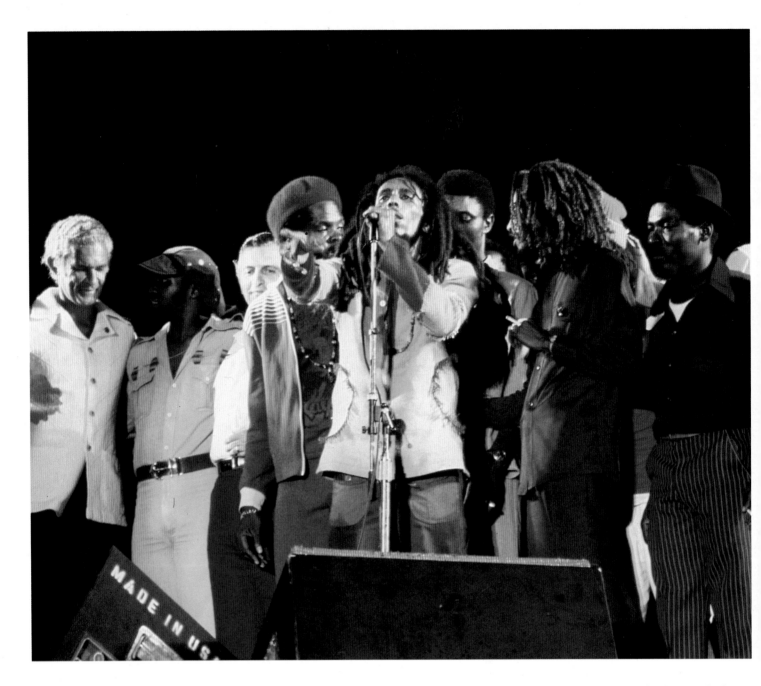

The accompanying video for 'Is This Love' was shot in home video style at a children's birthday party. Marley, surrounded by children of all races, was portrayed as a Pied Piper.

In mid-May, the Wailers started the US leg of their tour in Cleveland, Ohio, and went on to other dates in Ohio and in Wisconsin, Illinois, Minnesota, Michigan, Pennsylvania, New York, Washington DC, parts of Canada and finally Massachusetts.

Just before his sold-out June shows at New York's Madison Square Garden, Bob was honored by the United Nations. At the Waldorf-Astoria he was awarded the Third World Peace Medal. The New York shows in June were runaway successes and were widely photographed by the now Marley-hungry media.

Then it was off to Europe, where the band played in nine countries. A sold-out show at the Pavilion in Paris was recorded and released months later by Island as a double album called *Babylon By Bus*.

Although the band didn't choose the album title, it was ironically reflective of their current situation. They had an all-consuming touring schedule through countries whose governments the Rastas had derisively called 'Babylonian,' or oppressive towards their people.

TOP: **United symbolically in the colors of the rainbow: Marley, the Wailers and two of Jamaica's prime ministers, Manley and Seaga.**

RIGHT: **Marley speaks at the Waldorf-Astoria Hotel in New York City in June 1978.**

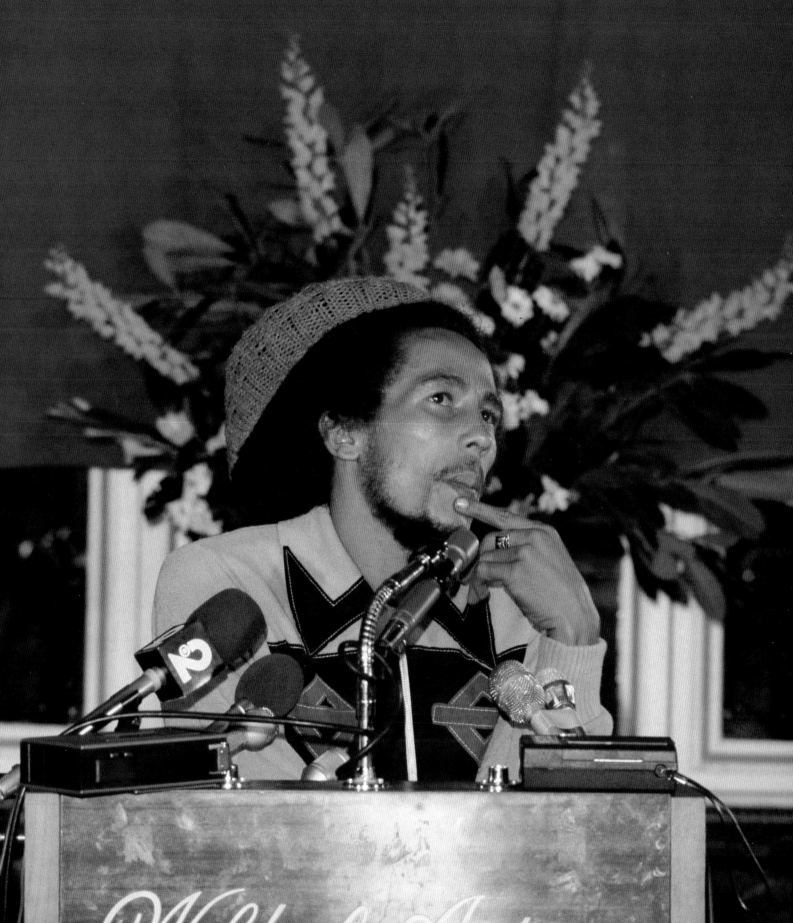

After a month in Europe, the band returned to North America to play dates in Vancouver, Canada, and the American west coast. During their appearance in Burbank, California, on 21 July, Peter Tosh joined the Wailers during the finale. Within the week, the band was down South making up the Exodus tour dates from the previous year.

When they returned, albeit briefly, to Jamaica, Bob got together with Lee Perry to record some new tracks including 'Burn Down Babylon' and 'Give Thanks and Praise.' Bob and the Wailers then departed for Australia, New Zealand and Japan, where they were a great success. With this tour, the Wailers' international superstar status was secured.

In September 1978, Peter Tosh was beaten by police. There was some speculation that it was a retaliatory attack for his anti-police comments at the One Love Peace Concert. His hand was broken and he was left cut and bruised.

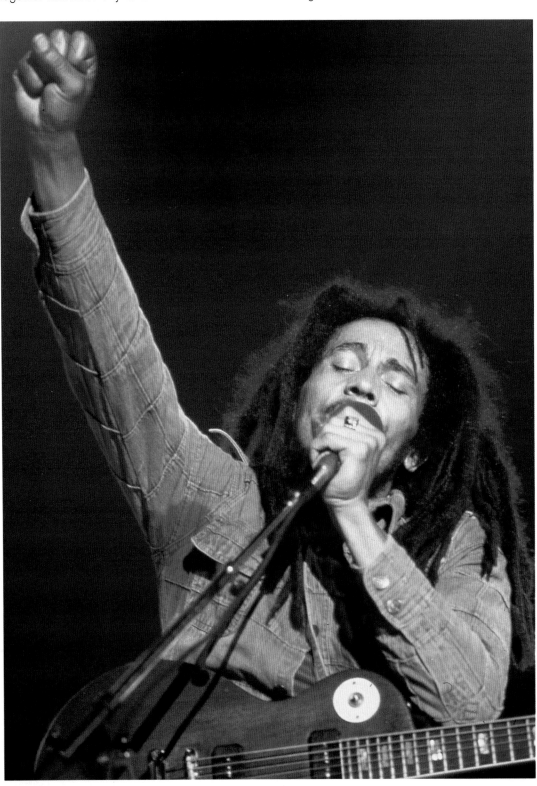

THESE PAGES: **Bob Marley's impassioned performances were legendary. These photos are from the Paris concert in 1978.**

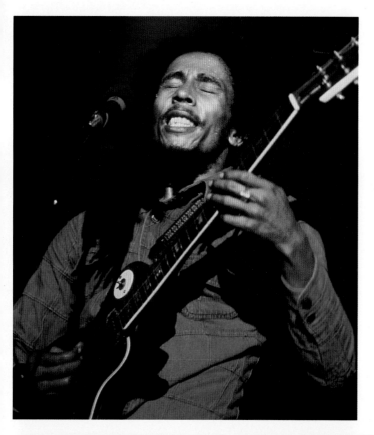

By this time, the Kaya tour was over and Marley had secured his visa to fulfil a dream: to travel to Africa. He visited Haile Selassie's homeland, Ethiopia, and then went on to Rhodesia, which would soon become Zimbabwe. Finally, Marley had a chance to explore the African roots of which he sang so vehemently. During his visit, he stayed on a religious commune and wrote.

When he returned to Jamaica, he was laden with new material and began to record at the newly constructed Tuff Gong studios at 56 Hope Road. However, the year 1979 would be a painful one for Marley. In February, Massop was found murdered in Jamaica, and later in the year Perry was hospitalized in Kingston after a nervous breakdown. The truce was long over, and guns and anguish still spoke the loudest in the ghetto.

Bob was an absolute musical perfectionist at this point, and he transformed his physical and spiritual pain into passionate, motivational music. For the next six months, he and the Wailers recorded what would become their ninth album for Island, *Survival*. It would include 'Zimbabwe,' 'Africa Unite,' 'Babylon System,' and the title track, 'Survival.'

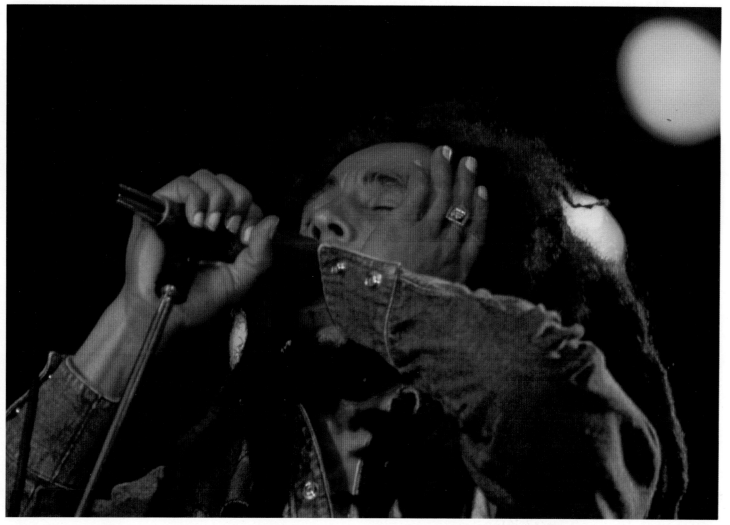

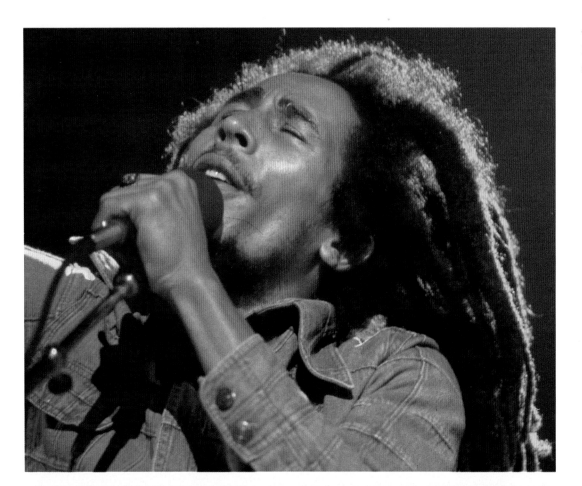

THESE PAGES: **More scenes of Bob Marley and the Wailers in concert, 1978.**

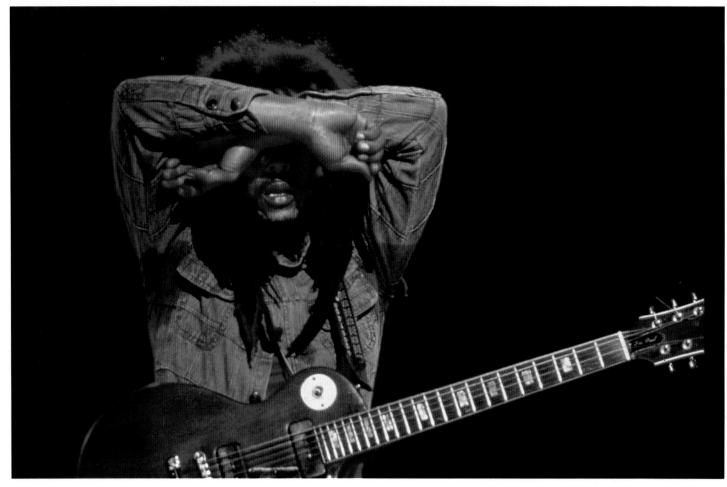

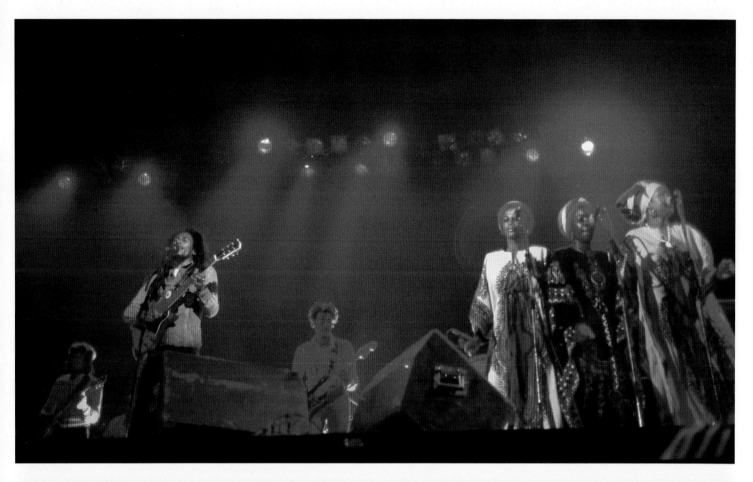

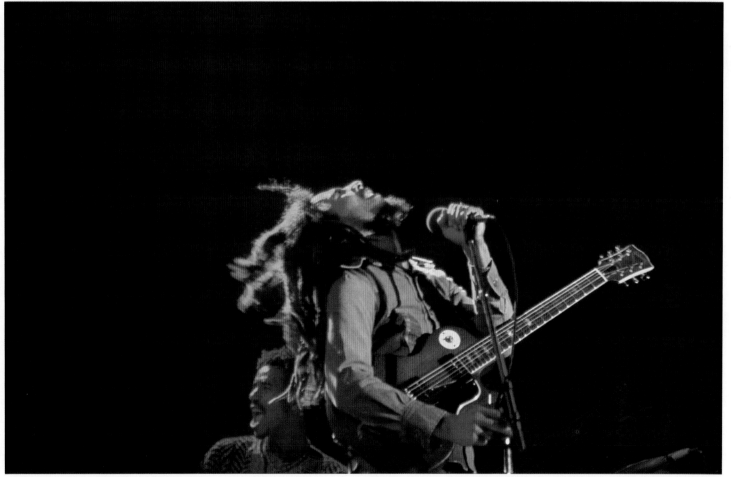

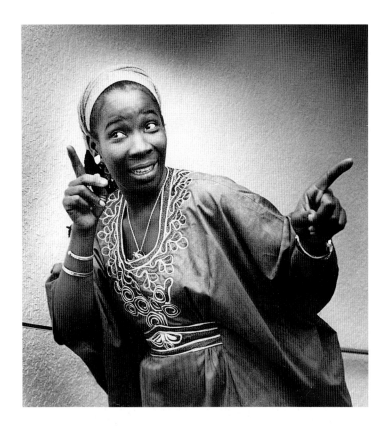

Despite his exhaustion following the worldwide gigs, he committed his talents to Africa. In Zimbabwe, a war between the black nationalists and an oppressive white minority government had been raging to the extent that a small nuclear device had been detonated to try to intimidate the guerrillas. Undaunted, the guerrillas had embraced Marley's 'Zimbabwe' as their inspirational battle hymn and were fighting tooth and nail for their country. When the independence-minded guerrillas had won, they arranged for a concert to be held in celebration. Once again, 17 April proved to be a significant day for Marley, as it had two years earlier: Marley and the Wailers were invited to perform in Zimbabwe on that date. The concert, held at Rufaro Stadium in Harare Township, formed a big part of the celebrations in the newly independent African state.

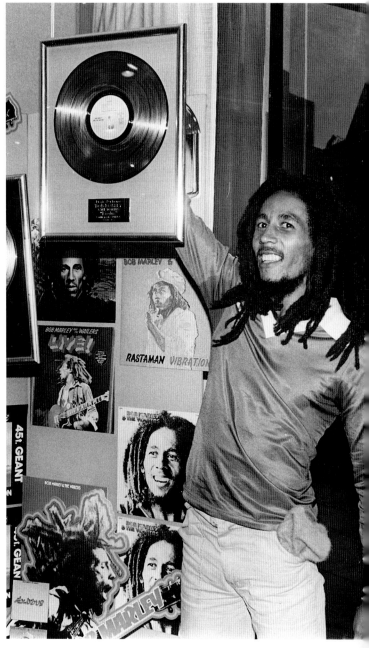

In July, Tuff Gong sponsored a night during Reggae Sunsplash II, a huge music festival. The Wailers performed to an ecstatic crowd. At the end of the night, Marley's two sons, Ziggy and Steve, danced onstage with their mother and father. Later that month, the band flew to Boston and played at a concert held to raise money for the 'liberation of Africa.' Marley was in rare form for that concert – some say it was his best live performance ever.

Also during that year, 'The Melody Makers,' Bob and Rita's children, marked their debut with one of Bob's compositions, 'Children Playing in the Streets.' It was released under the Tuff Gong label, and the proceeds benefitted the UN Children's Fund.

On 24 September, the Wailers performed at a benefit for Rasta children in Kingston. Soon after, they travelled to the United States to begin the Survival tour.

On this tour, Bob hoped he would reach the black audiences which had so far eluded him in the United States. During the tour, Stevie Wonder performed with them at the Black Music Association Convention in Philadelphia. Bob Marley and the Wailers also played several nights at the famed Apollo Theater in Harlem, Marcus Garvey's old stomping ground.

It was to be another extensive US tour, lasting almost two months and covering the East and West coasts, then moving on to the Caribbean. Unfortunately, this time Bob's reduced energy level due to the encroachment of the cancer cells left him lagging behind. He kept writing new material, but left a good deal of the promotion to the band.

LEFT: Rita, proud matriarch of the Marley clan, also had a well-established recording career of her own.

BELOW LEFT: Bob celebrates the success of *Exodus* in Paris, 1978.

RIGHT: Weary, yet still filled with passion, Bob Marley sings to the crowd in 1978.

BELOW: The Wailers play before a backdrop decorated with the illustration used on the cover of the *Uprising* album, 1980.

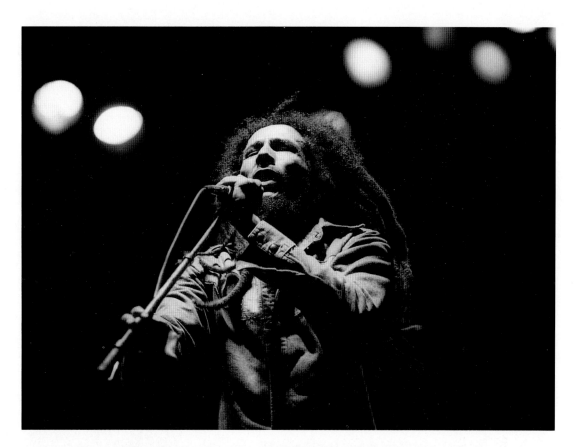

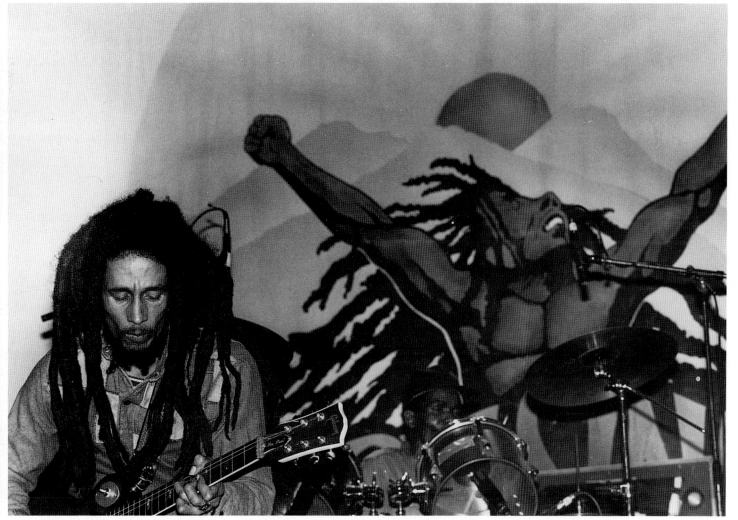

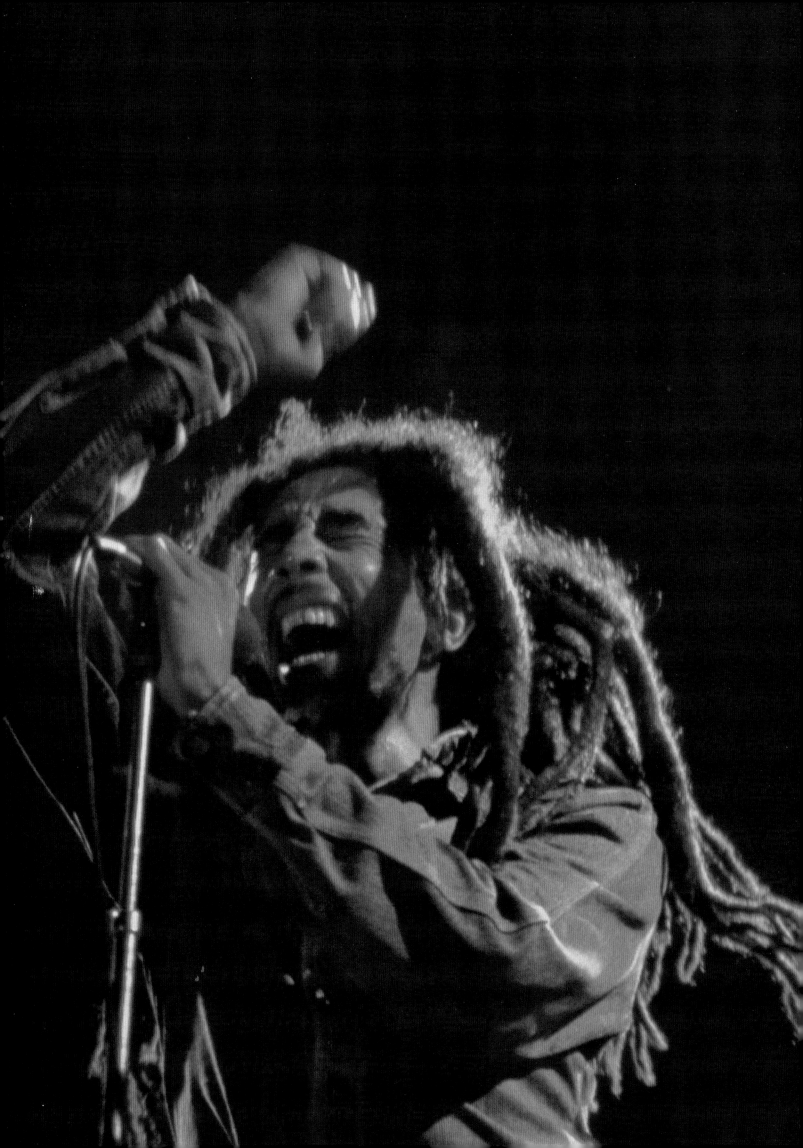

THESE PAGES: Scenes from the
Wailers' European tour, 1980.

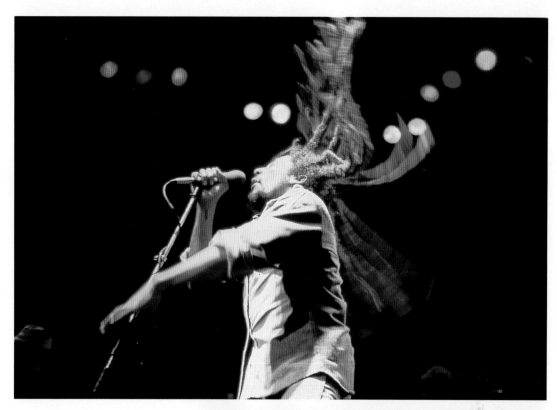

Upon their return from Africa, the band members were
reminded of their own country's political strife when they heard
Bucky Marshall was found shot to death in Brooklyn.

The band's tenth album, *Uprising*, was released in May 1980,
and again the American tour was targeted toward the black
audience. The illustration on the album cover depicted Marley,
clenched fists held triumphantly overhead. It was successful
commercially upon its release.

Unfortunately, the dawn of 1980 brought the violence of another
election year in Jamaica. By the time the election was over in
October, nearly 700 would be dead. Once again, although not as
significantly, reggae music was used during the pre-election
campaign. Both parties used the same two Marley compositions,
without his permission, to promote their campaigns: 'Coming In
From the Cold' and 'Bad Card,' both from *Uprising*.

The maddening concert pace began in Switzerland this time
and covered twelve European countries. In August, the band
retreated to Miami to avoid Jamaica's turmoils and to relax. Bob's
health was clearly deteriorating, but he got the go-ahead from his
doctor to continue the tour. The US tour started in mid-
September in Boston.

When the band arrived in New York to perform with the
Commodores at Madison Square Garden, the band members
were, oddly, put up in two separate hotels. Rita immediately knew
something was wrong, because great efforts were made to isolate
Bob from the band.

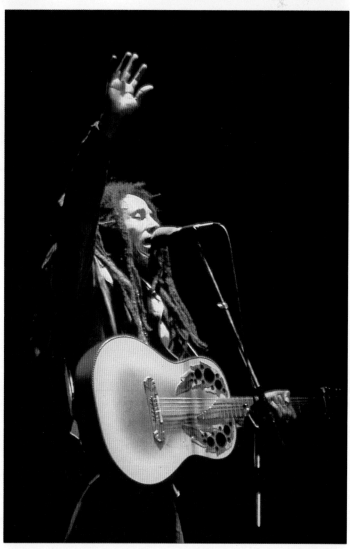

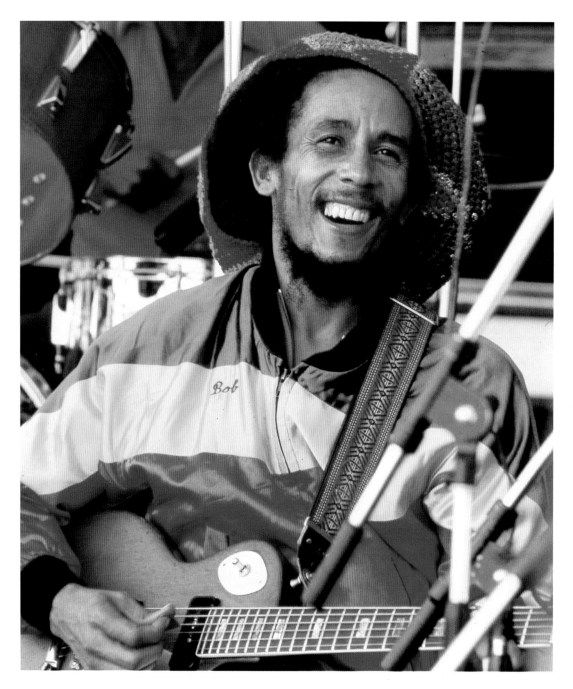

During one of the New York concerts, Bob nearly blacked out. The following morning, 21 September, he decided to go for a run with Skilly Cole in Central Park. He collapsed and was carried back to the hotel. Within days, Marley was told he had a brain tumor and had suffered a stroke in the park. He was also told he wouldn't live another month. Everyone, and most of all Bob, was shocked.

Rita wasn't informed until later, because she and the I-Threes had flown ahead as instructed to the next city. Despite his illness, Bob insisted on going on to Pittsburgh for the next show.

That night, Rita had a vivid dream that Bob, who had lost all of his hair, was talking to her through a wire fence, telling her how sick he was. The next day, when Rita actually saw his withered skeleton, she began insisting that the tour be cancelled. Bob prevailed and played a brilliant show that night at the Stanley Theater in Pittsburgh.

Rita called Diane Jobson, Bob's trusted lawyer and advisor, and Danny Sims, to ensure that the tour was stopped. On 23 September, it was reported that Bob Marley was suffering from 'exhaustion' and the Tuff Gong Uprising tour was cancelled.

Bob was flown from Miami to New York's Memorial Sloan-Kettering Cancer Center where he was fully diagnosed as having brain, lung and stomach cancer. He was flown back to Miami where, on 4 November, he was baptized as Berhane Selassie in the Ethiopian Orthodox Church, a Christian church, at Rita's suggestion.

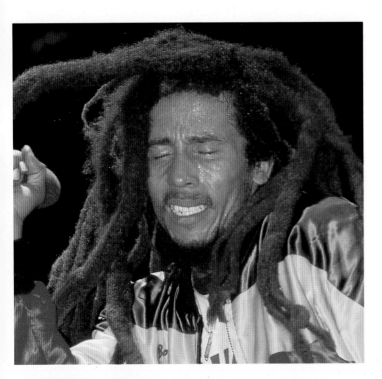

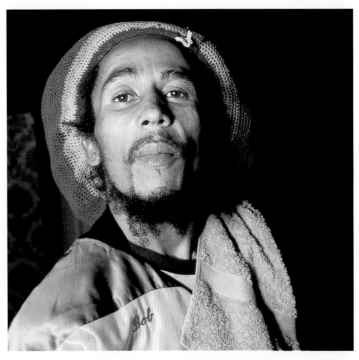

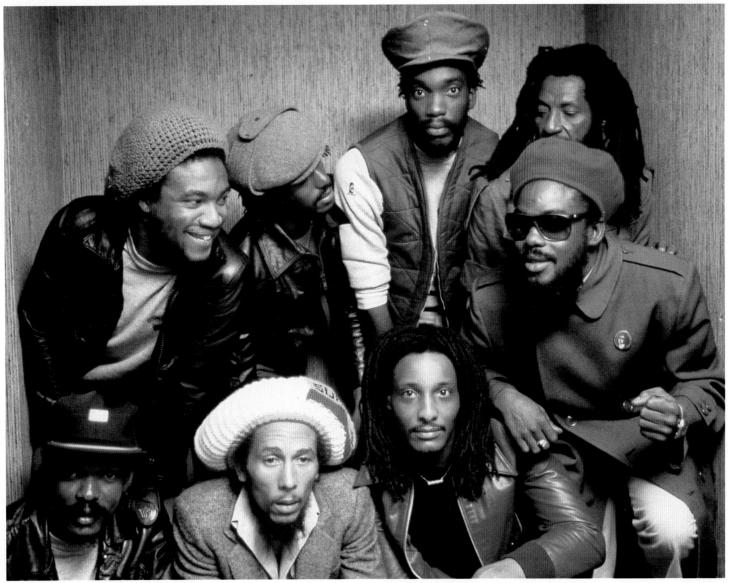

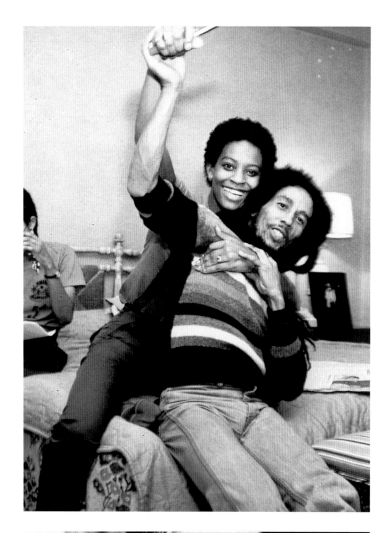

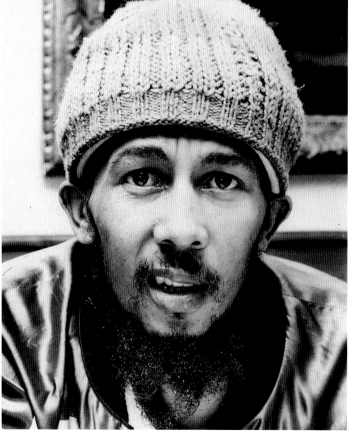

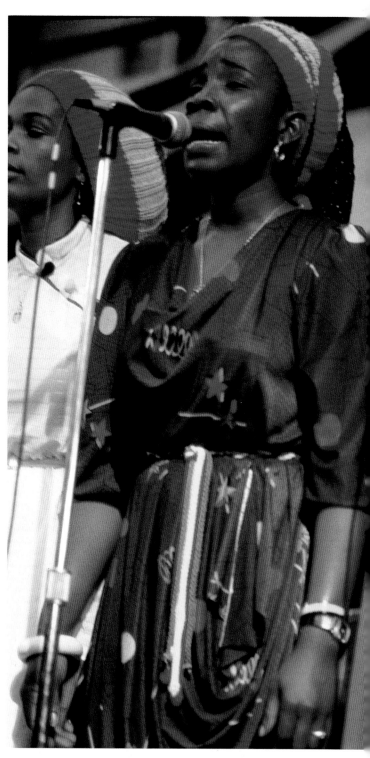

TOP LEFT: The last known photo taken of Bob in New York City, with an unidentified woman, in 1981.

LEFT: Bob smiles weakly at the Issels Clinic in Germany after losing his dreadlocks to radiation therapy.

Five days later, in a last ditch effort to prolong his life, Bob was flown to a controversial treatment center in Bavaria, Germany. Dr Josef Issels ran the clinic, and had been successful in treating 'terminal' cases before.

Bob celebrated his thirty-sixth birthday in February 1981 at

the clinic. When he arrived, Marley had lost his hair but now he seemed to be gaining strength and his hair was growing back. He was, however, still losing weight. It wasn't until May that his demise was evident. On 11 May 1981, a full six months later, Bob Marley died. His wife and mother were at his bedside.

Prophet Gad had insisted prior to Marley's death that he should become the owner of the Lion of Judah ring. Mysteriously, however, the ring disappeared and hasn't been seen since. Bob's mother claimed it went back from whence it came.

Marley's funeral in Jamaica was fit for a king. Hundreds of thousands turned out for the celebration, for Marley was at last living completely with 'Jah Rastafari.'

LEFT: **Rita Marley sings at Bob's funeral with the I-Threes. He died on 11 May 1981.**

BELOW: **Thousands lined the motorcade route leading into the Kingston stadium where the funeral was held. Marley was buried in St Ann parish, the place of his birth.**

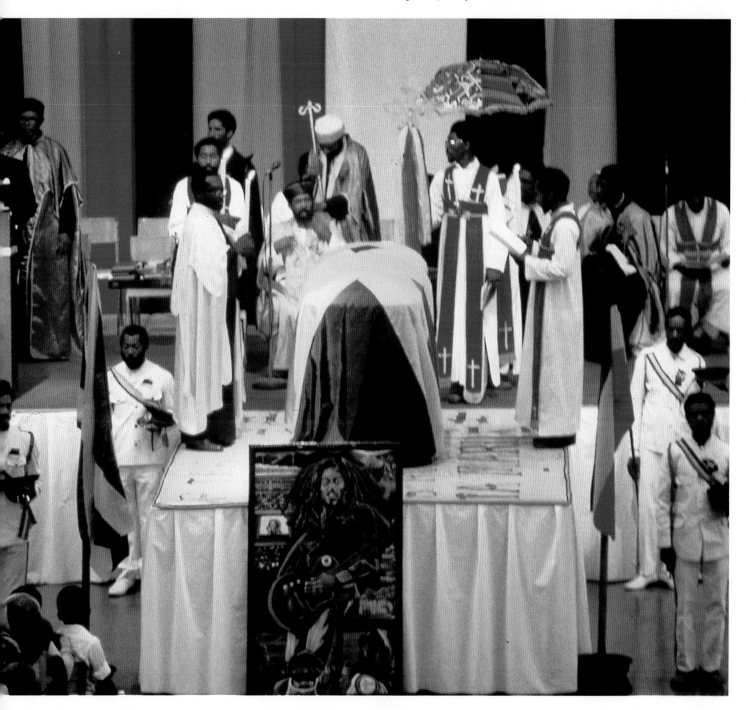

LEGEND
1981 - Present

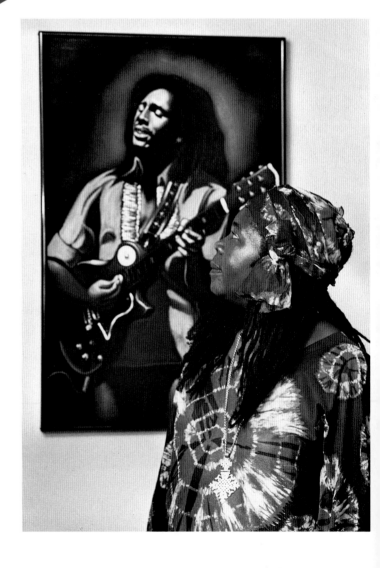

RIGHT: **Cedella Booker admires a portrait of her son Bob in her office.**

When Bob Marley died, at the young age of 36, some believed that the age of reggae music was over. But they failed to notice that he had become a legend, and a legend's influence never dies.

Musicians have turned to Marley's music time and time again for inspiration. Paul Simon, Eric Clapton, the Police, and Stevie Wonder are just a few of the American musicians who were strongly influenced by Marley's brand of reggae. Reggae musicians still do well in the United States and abroad although none have attained the larger-than-life reputation of Marley. However, such groups as Black Uhuru, Steel Pulse and Linton Kwesi Johnson are continuing his legacy.

The 'roots' reggae that Marley and his contemporaries played has evolved into different forms throughout the years. Today's reggae has been recreated, as most music has, in a new form.

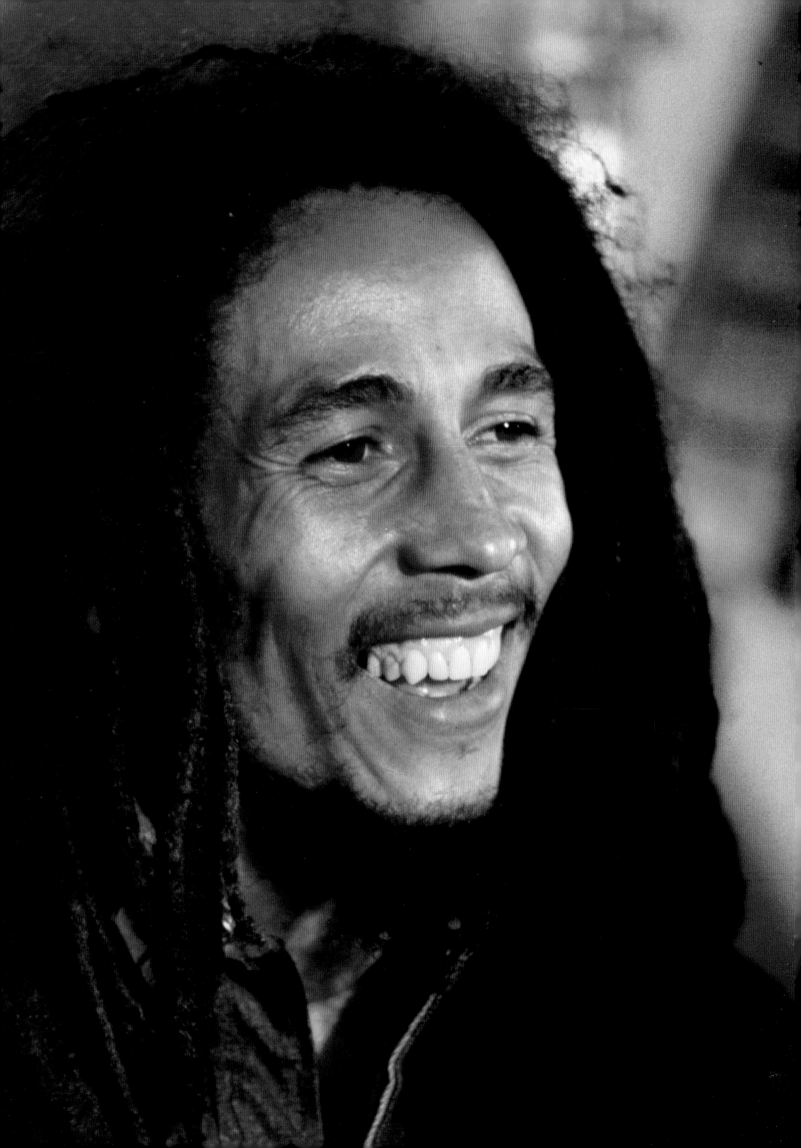

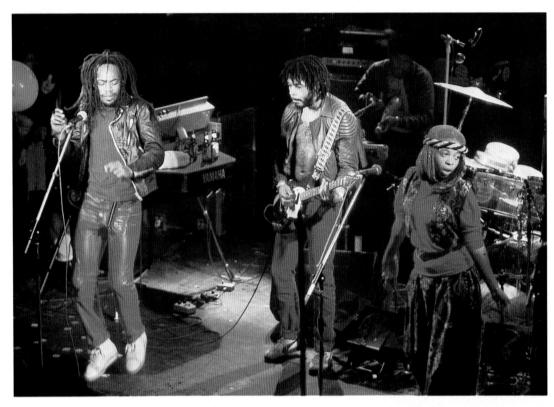

LEFT: **Black Uhuru, loyal to the roots-reggae sound, has consistently topped Billboard's World Chart and was nominated for a Grammy.**

BELOW: **Bob Marley's message is as relevant today as it was when he was alive.**

In the summer of 1992, Jimmy Cliff said of the metamorphosis of popular music: '. . . the rock and roll that Chuck Berry or Elvis Presley played is a different rock and roll today but it's still called rock and roll. So music is a t'ing that changes all the time, so the reggae that was in the sixties and the seventies, even the eighties is a different reggae now than in the nineties. That's music, that's the nature of music. It changes with the people you know, it's changing now . . . .'

The latest dancehall craze is a combination of reggae and rap. Musicians such as Shabba Ranks, Mad Cobra and Super Cat are responsible for the popularization of the music. These artists, not unlike their ska and rock steady counterparts in the early 1960s, sing about girls and guns. Their experiences also come from tough, ghetto streets.

These musicians have captured the audience Marley craved while he was alive: black Americans. Bob aimed his lyrical genius at this audience, but somehow failed to capture it. For some reason, his audience was almost always predominantly white. The special message he tried to give black Americans was a history lesson that would give them a sense of their roots: who they were, and where they came from.

One of the messages in music today is one that Marley scorned during his lifetime: violence. Although many contemporary songs are not specifically violence-oriented, they do not culturally inform or motivate. They do not give 'upliftment,' as Marley would say.

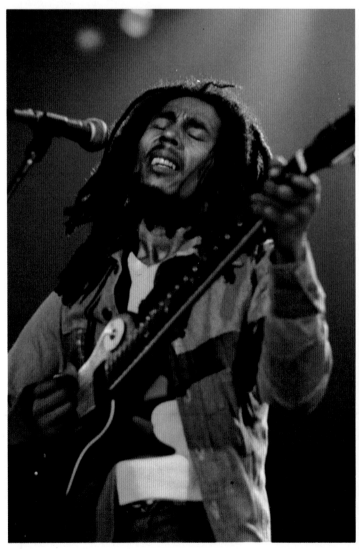

RIGHT: Jimmy Cliff is now combining traditional reggae beats with Brazilian samba drums and electronic instruments.

BELOW: Steel Pulse still retains the original roots-reggae sound despite the popularity of dancehall-style music.

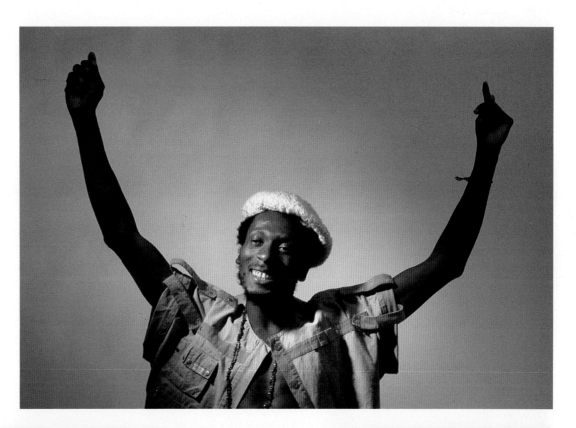

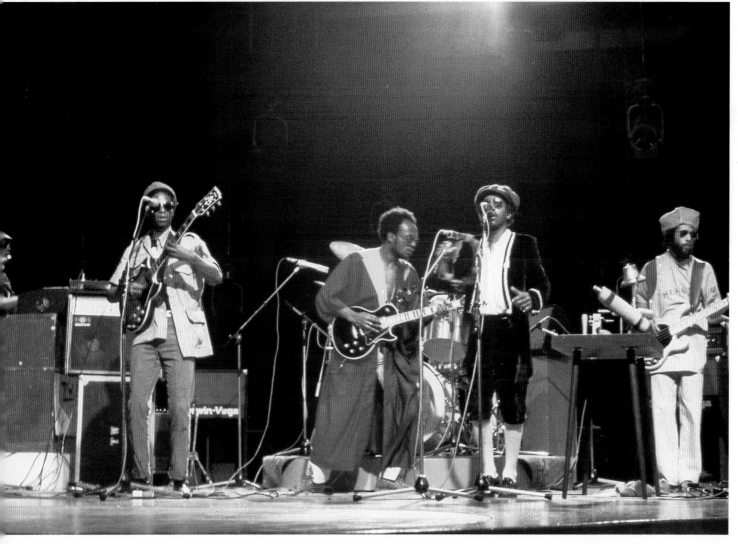

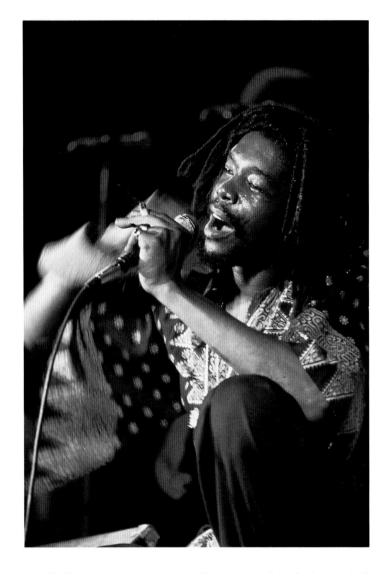

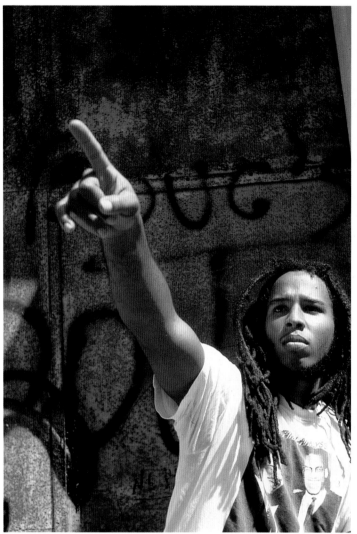

Unlike 'roots' reggae, recognition came quickly for its musical offspring. In 1992, Shabba Ranks won a Grammy for *As Raw as Ever*. It was the first time a reggae album had ever topped *Billboard* magazine's R&B charts. He won a Grammy again in 1993, for his album *X-tra Naked*.

Jimmy Cliff was able to shed some light on the phenomenon from a 'roots' reggae perspective. 'The DJ has become a phenomenal form now. I don't t'ink it has a lot of conscious message as far as like consciousness of your culture, origin, now as it did then, but maybe that's not the spirit of the people now.'

Cliff feels that even in its present form, people can relate to the music: 'It still has an impact 'cause it's danceable. It's a different sound, a different rhythm. But the conscious message of culture, of origin, and upliftment . . . I don't think it's carrying that now.'

In Jamaica, music has long been a way to spread the news. Ska was the tense music of the rudies, rock steady was for lovers and reggae for spiritual rebels. In the 1992 video *Time Will Tell* released by Island Visual Arts, Marley says, 'Reggae music is people music, it's news,' and 'Reggae is a music created by Rasta people.

ABOVE LEFT: **Former original Wailer Peter Tosh had an active solo career until he was shot and killed in Jamaica in 1987.**

ABOVE: **Ziggy Marley helps to carry on his father's legacy.**

ABOVE RIGHT: **Rita Marley fought the Jamaican courts for ten years to gain control of the Marley estate.**

FAR RIGHT ABOVE: **Thanks to performers such as Sinead O'Connor, Bob Marley's message is still being heard.**

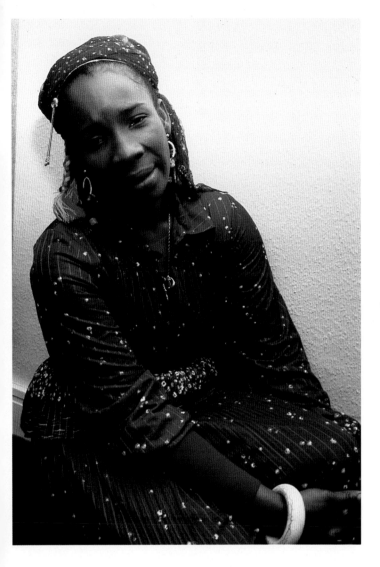

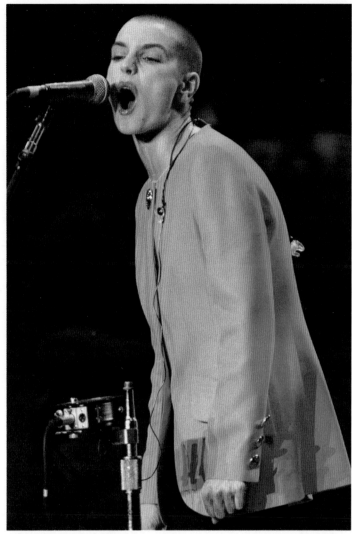

And it carry earth force . . . a people rhythm, it's a rhythm of people working, people moving.' Obviously the news has changed.

Marley's message, however, remains relevant. During his life, he preached equality for all, regardless of the color of their skin. Perhaps in unifying people he united himself, both black and white. He spoke of the injustice of oppression of any kind, especially economic and spiritual. He loudly demanded respect for people's rights to a good life, during which they should be allowed to find out who they are and where they came from.

A dozen years after his death, Marley still wins new converts every year, and his legacy has been continued by his wife and children. Rita has a contract with Shenachie Records, and 'Ziggy Marley and the Melody Makers' have met with moderate success. In 1985 the group was nominated for a Grammy Award. Ziggy also looks amazingly like his father.

Upon his death, Marley refused to leave a will, believing it was a symbol of 'Babylon.' Rita was accused of embezzling money from the estate by J Louis Byles, the Jamaican court-appointed lawyer, during the 1980s. Rita claimed, since the estate was

legally half hers and her children's, that it was her right to divert particular funds. She argued that she could not steal from herself. After a ten-year legal tangle, involving royalty rights for his band members and trusts for his numerous illegitimate children, Rita was acquitted in 1992. Settlements were made with all the other parties.

Despite the 'Babylonian' realities, roots reggae is still played to sell-out crowds in summer festivals such as the Summer Sunsplash, Reggae Festival, and the World Beat tours.

In the US, Sunday nights have become reggae nights at many metropolitan bars and Marley's music is still played frequently on the radio.

In 1992, Sinead O'Connor, an Irish singer, performed Marley's 'War' a capella on the television program 'Saturday Night Live.' A baffled crowd watched her end her performance by tearing up a picture of the Pope and saying, 'Fight the real enemy.' Despite O'Connor's performance, the words of Marley's song, taken from a speech given by Haile Selassie I, are still relevant today. Racial tensions continue to ignite Kingston and

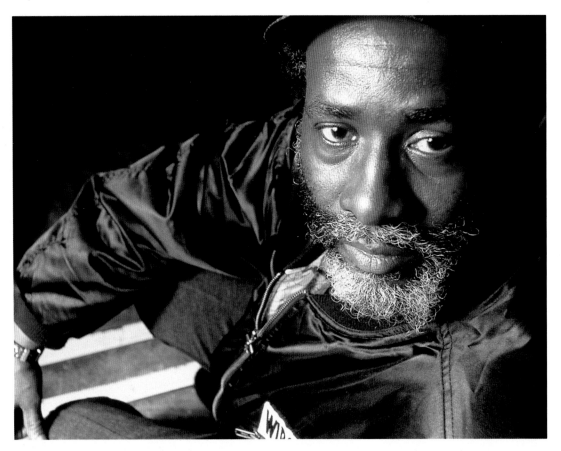

LEFT: Burning Spear headlined with Jimmy Cliff during the World Beat '92 Tour and is currently signed to Mango Records, a division of Island Records.

BELOW: All of the Marleys, including Bob's mother, are active in the recording industry as singers and songwriters. Shown left to right: daughter Cedella, son Julian, wife Rita, son Stevie, and mother Cedella.

BELOW RIGHT: Bob Marley's music continues to be an inspiration to generations of listeners and musicians.

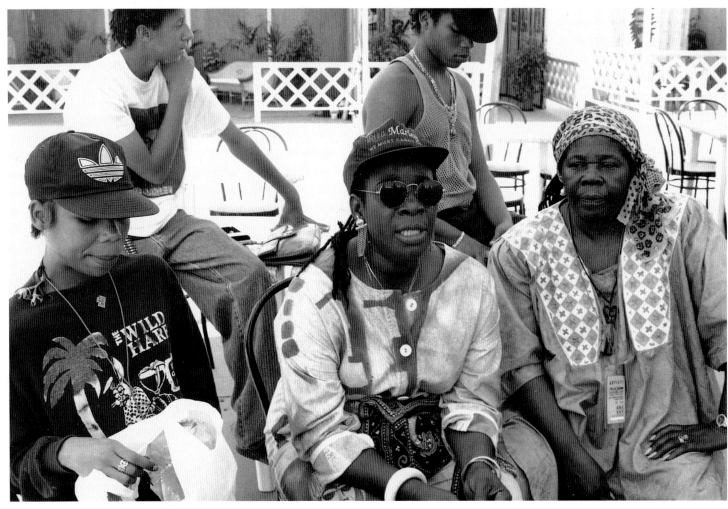

impoverished ghettos all over the world. Conditions have actually gotten worse since Marley was alive.

Commercially, Marley also lives on. Shops carry Marley memorabilia: T-shirts, hats, keychains and posters, some of which include the Lion of Judah symbol or Rasta colors. Many shop owners who sell the merchandise claim that Marley items remain some of their most popular.

In 1992, Tuff Gong, a division of Island records, released a compilation of Marley's work spanning the length of his 19-year career called 'Songs of Freedom.' Tuff Gong and Island Visual Arts also released the video that same year. A magazine called *Tuff Gong* that will espouse Marley's philosophy and discuss his work, heritage and identity, is also in the works. The Robert Marley Foundation and the Bob Marley Museum now occupy his old residence at 56 Hope Road.

Bob Marley wanted everyone to be free, and he used his gift towards that end. He sent a new type of music, reggae, across the water and the airwaves where it could be exposed to millions of people. Through this music he sent a powerful message – one of anti-racism, peace and love for all. He was a spiritually driven man who felt he had to fulfill his calling. He was charismatic and mysterious and captivated millions with his special brand of love – his music.

During 1992, the Jamaican Tourism Board used a cover version of Bob Marley's 'One Love' as its theme song. Television commercials for Jamaica stressed the beautiful lush green of the land and the peace, beauty and harmony of the people, who stand side by side, regardless of color. It's ironic that what is being advertised today as the perfect Jamaica is all Bob Marley ever wanted.

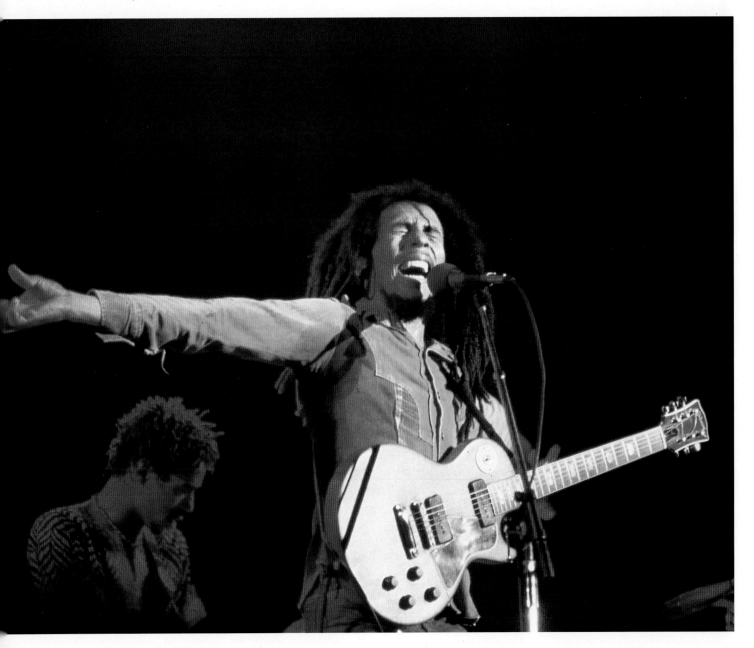

DISCOGRAPHY

The following Bob Marley albums are still being distributed:

Label	Title	Year	Label	Title	Year
Bella Musica	Bob Marley	1990		Exodus	1977
Columbia	Birth of a Legend	1990		Kaya	1978
	Early Music	1977		Babylon By Bus	1978
Cotillion	Chances Are	1981		Survival	1979
Epic Associated	Birth of a Legend (1963-66)	1990		Uprising	1980
Forlane	Saga, Volume I			Confrontation	1983
	Saga, Volume II	1991		Legend	1984
Garland	Reggae Roots			Rebel Music	1986
Heartbeat Records	One Love	1992		Talkin' Blues	1991
Island/Tuff Gong	Catch a Fire	1973		Songs of Freedom	1992
	Burnin'	1973	Pair	The Mighty Bob Marley	1989
	Natty Dread	1974		More of the Mighty Bob Marley	1990
	Live! Bob Marley & The Wailers		Special Music Company	Bob Marley At His Best	1989
	(at the Lyceum)	1975		Reggae Magic	
	Rastaman Vibration	1976			

RIGHT: Always an exciting performer, Bob Marley puts heart and soul into a concert during the Exodus tour, 1977.

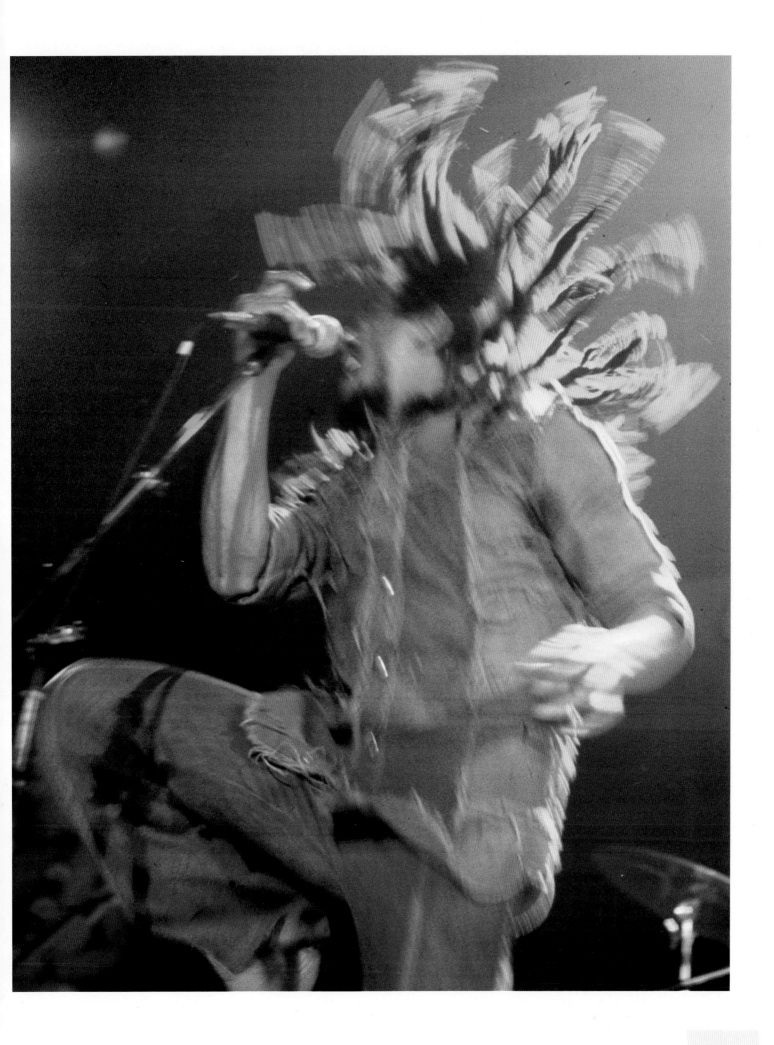

Index